DATE DUE

#45220 Highsmith Inc. 1-800-558-2110

A DICTIONARY OF DRUG ABUSE TERMS AND TERMINOLOGY

A DICTIONARY OF DRUG ABUSE TERMS AND TERMINOLOGY

Ernest L. Abel

Greenwood Press
Westport, Connecticut · London, England

Library of Congress Cataloging in Publication Data

Abel, Ernest L., 1943–
    A dictionary of drug abuse terms and terminology.

    Bibliography: p.
    Includes index.
    1. Drug abuse—Dictionaries.   I. Title.
HV5804.A23   1984   362.2′93′0321   83-22867
ISBN 0-313-24095-7 (lib. bdg.)

Library of Congress Catalog Card Number: 83-22867
ISBN: 0-313-24095-7

First published in 1984

Greenwood Press
A division of Congressional Information Service, Inc.
88 Post Road West
Westport, Connecticut 06881

Printed in the United States of America

10 9 8 7 6 5 4 3 2 1

Contents

Preface

This dictionary contains words and expressions dealing with drugs of abuse along with some technical terms that are frequently encountered in this context. Many of the terms relating to marihuana have been adopted from my previous text, *A Marihuana Dictionary*. The main difference between that book and the present one is that the former was concerned solely with marihuana and was presented on historical principles, that is, definitions were given and examples of such definitions were presented along with the dates and sources for such examples. In the present book, terms relating to marihuana constitute only a portion of the book, and no attempt has been made to present anything more than a cursory historical context for a few terms.

A major omission in the present book concerns words and expressions relating to alcohol and tobacco. The reason that this body of words has been omitted is that it numbers in the thousands and inclusion of some terms and not others would be completely arbitrary. Nevertheless, some of the most common terms relating to alcohol and tobacco have been noted.

Although comprehensive, this dictionary is by no means exhaustive. This is because this language is ephemeral and regional in nature. Many words and expressions disappear almost as soon as they are coined, and other terms are used in only one part of the country.

Entries are arranged alphabetically in the text. A detailed glossary that serves as another form of organization for this material is provided at the end of the text. A detailed bibliography has also been included.

Introduction

A major difficulty in discussing the language of drug abuse is that it covers such a wide territory. Drug abuse can take several forms, such as use of illicit drugs or misuse of medically approved drugs. In the context of drugs taken for their psychic effects, the drugs most frequently mentioned as responsible for drug-related hospital emergency visits include alcohol, Valium, marihuana, PCP, methaqualone, cocaine, heroin/morphine, aspirin, LSD, pentazocine, amphetamine, flurazepam, codeine, acetaminophen, haloperidol, phenobarbital, and propoxyphene.

Alcohol used in combination with other drugs accounts for the majority of such visits. The frequency of visits for the other drugs occurs roughly in the order they are cited above. Obviously emergency room visits do not reflect drug abuse patterns in general, but they do reflect such patterns to some extent. The different categories of drugs are also interesting since these include alcohol, tranquilizers (e.g., Valium), marihuana, hallucinogens (e.g., PCP), nonbarbiturate sedatives (e.g., methaqualone), barbiturate sedatives (e.g., phenobarbital), amphetamines, and narcotics, as well as nonnarcotic painkillers such as aspirin. There is in essence no single type of drug abuser.

Drug abuse can be further broken down into male/female differences. Males, for instance, are more likely than females to use alcohol in combination with other drugs and to use marihuana, PCP, methaqualone, cocaine, and narcotics, whereas females are more likely to be abusers of Valium and aspirin.

Another breakdown can be made along racial lines. Whites are more likely to be abusers of alcohol in combination with other drugs, Valium, and methaqualone, whereas blacks are more likely to be abusers of narcotics and PCP.

The point is that everyone belongs to many subcultures, each of which has its own language that stems from his or her own experiences. The drug abuser whose drug of choice is medically sanctioned is unlikely to share the experiences of the drug abuser whose drug of choice is illegal.

A subculture is a group of people that is in many ways different from the rest of society. The drug abuse subculture is one that shares common needs, interests, attitudes, behavioral patterns, and pressures from within itself and from the dominant culture, involving drugs. As such, the drug abuse subculture has developed its own special language to express these special concerns. But as I have already pointed out, there is no single drug culture but rather several different drug subcultures. Yet even though these subcultures differ from one another, they do share a common concern, and sometimes an obsession, with drug use, and their special languages tend to borrow from one another. While these special languages in many ways overlap the language of the dominant culture, they are constantly developing new terms or giving meaning to already existent words.

In the case of illegal drug use, buying and using drugs has had to be and still is very secretive. A key element in this clandestine effort is the development and refining of a special language—a lingo—by which users can communicate with one another and identify who is a user and who is not.

Lingos or argots, as students of language call them, are not developed solely to hide behind. Another important reason for their evolution is to foster group solidarity and cohesiveness. Many of those who use a particular lingo derive pleasure from it. They take pride in using it and judge others by their knowledge of it. This seems more particularly true for users of "soft" drugs than for users of "hard" drugs.

A lingo promotes camaraderie and cohesiveness because it reflects and embodies the thinking and life-styles of the group. Like all slang, however, the lingo of drug abuse is constantly changing. As soon as various terms become widely known to and used by the public, they are dropped and are replaced by new terms. This is because the members of the subculture may feel they are losing their unique identity as their language becomes known and adopted by the dominant culture. The diffusion of language from the subculture of "hard" drugs to that of "soft" drugs reflects assimilation of these two subcultures. Likewise, the diffusion of the "soft" drug subculture to the dominant culture also reflects an increasing tendency for the dominant culture to adopt the behavior of the "soft" drug subculture. It is this threat of loss of identity through loss of language that motivates adoption of new words and new meanings for older words. But even with the ephemeral quality of much of the lingo, there always seems to be a core of terms that is perpetuated through generations as if it were a cultural heirloom.

Drug abuse lingo seems to intrigue both scholars and the general public. Scholars are fascinated by this language within a language because it offers new insights into an American subculture. The general public seems just as fascinated by the colorful language, as witnessed by the many pop songs, movies, magazines, and books containing such jargon. Often these terms are used without any explanation on the assumption that they are so well known that no explanation is needed. At other times, however, it is very difficult to know what is being said without being a member of the drug culture.

One of the questions that frequently pops up whenever anyone talks about the language of drug abuse is the origin of such terms. Unfortunately, the etymology of many of these words is lost. In some cases they have been borrowed from other subcultures. For instance, the user of illegal drugs is often forced into other criminal activity or forced to associate with criminals either on the street or in jail. Such encounters invariably result in a broadening of the drug abuser's lexicon. The drug abuser also uses words from the other subcultures of which he or she is a member and often in so doing gives those words new and specialized meanings. The etymology of most slang words, however, is almost impossible to determine.

A DICTIONARY OF DRUG ABUSE TERMS AND TERMINOLOGY

A

A 1. Acid, referring to LSD. 2. Amphetamines.

A Boot Under the influence of a drug.

AA Alcoholics Anonymous.

Ab Abscess from using an infected needle for injection of drugs, usually narcotics.

Abbott Nembutal, a barbiturate. Derived from manufacturer's name, Abbott Laboratories.

Abe Five-dollar purchase of drugs. From the picture of Abraham Lincoln on the five-dollar bill.

A-bomb *See* Atom Bomb.

Absolute alcohol 100 percent ethyl alcohol. *See* Alcohol.

Absorption Passage of substances such as drugs across bodily membranes.

Abstinence Avoidance of a form of behavior such as drug taking. Abstinence may result in withdrawal.

Abstinence syndrome Withdrawal reaction from a drug. *See* Withdrawal.

Abuse, drug Nontherapeutic use of drugs to the point where it affects the health of the individual or impacts adversely on others. The term is very subjective.

Abuse potential Likelihood of a particular substance being used inappropriately and to excess. *See* Drug abuse.

Acapulco Gold Potent form of marihuana originating near the tropical resort town in Mexico, golden brown in color.

Acapulco Gold papers Cigarette papers made from marihuana fiber.

Acapulco Red Like Acapulco Gold except the color is reddish brown.

Ace 1. Marihuana cigarette. 2. One-year jail term. 3. One dollar. 4. To cheat someone. 5. PCP.

Acetomorphine Derivative of opium.

Acetone Volatile solvent used as fingernail polish remover and in plastic cements. Sometimes used as a volatile inhalant.

Acetylmethadol Narcotic analgesic. *See* LAAM.

Acid LSD.

Acid Dropper User of LSD.

Acid Freak Frequent user of LSD.

Acid Funk LSD-induced depression.

Acid Head *Same as* Acid Freak.

Acid Lab Place where LSD is made.

Acid Pad Place where LSD is taken.

Acid Party Party at which LSD is taken.

Acid Test Ability to take LSD and experience no adverse effects.

Ack Ack To smoke heroin by placing it on the tip of a burning cigarette.

ACM *See* American Council on Marihuana and Other Psychoactive Drugs.

ACT *See* Alliance for Cannabis Therapeutics.

Action 1. Any activity. 2. A "happening." 3. Purchase or sale of drugs.

Active ingredient, principal Substance in a drug or plant primarily responsible for its psychoactive effects. For example, the principal active ingredient in opium is morphine.

Acute Of short duration, often involving an intense response; opposite of chronic.

Ad 1. Narcotics addict. 2. PCP.

ADAMHA *See* Alcohol, Drug Abuse, and Mental Health Administration. The agency under the U.S. Department of Health and Human Services that oversees the National Institute on Drug Abuse (NIDA), the National Institute on Alcohol Abuse and Alcoholism (NIAAA), and the National Institute on Mental Health (NIMH).

Adaptation *See* Tolerance.

Addict Individual with a compulsive need to use a particular substance. Generally used in reference to narcotics users.

Addiction Condition resulting from repeated drug use, consisting of a compulsive urge to keep using the drug and to get it by any means, a tendency to increase the amount being used, and a physical dependence that results in withdrawal following abstinence. *See also* Dependence.

Addiction liability Substance that can become addicting.

Addiction Research Foundation Canadian agency involved in research and treatment of drug-related problems. Located in Toronto.

Addiction-prone personality Individual with a special personality characteristic that renders him or her inclined to use drugs in order to deal with personal problems.

Additive effect Additive impact of two or more substances taken together. *See also* Potentiation; Synergism.

Administration route Means by which a drug is introduced into the body. This can be by swallowing, inhalation, absorption through the skin or other surface membranes, or directly by injection into the blood or muscles or under the skin.

Adulteration Dilution of a drug with either an inert material to add bulk or some more potent material to create a greater effect.

Adverse reaction Unpleasant reaction to a drug. Includes anxiety, paranoia, sense of loss of control, dysphoria.

Affect Emotional feeling or response.

Afghani Potent hashish or marihuana from Afghanistan.

African Black Potent hashish from Africa, blackish in color.

Aftercare Care and treatment of an individual after release from a drug abuse program. Designed to help integrate the individual into society and prevent return to drug use.

Afternoon Farmer Opium smoker who does not keep appointments.

Agonies Withdrawal symptoms associated with narcotics use.

Agonist Pharmacological term referring to a substance that binds with a drug receptor to produce a drug-related response. *See* Antagonist.

A-head 1. Frequent user of amphetamines. 2. Frequent user of LSD.

AIDS Acquired immune deficiency syndrome. Lowering of body's immune defenses. Associated with intravenous drug administration.

Aimies Amphetamines.

AIP Afghanistan, Iran, Pakistan. A "Golden Triangle," source of opium eventually converted into heroin.

Airplane *See* Jefferson Airplane.

Alcohol Class of chemical compounds that share a particular structure. Ethyl alcohol, also known as ethanol or grain alcohol is a colorless liquid that is the principal intoxicating substance in wine, beer, and liquors. The concentration of alcohol in beer is about 4 percent; in table wine, about 12 percent; in fortified wine, about 20 percent; and in distilled spirits, about 50 percent.

Contrary to popular belief, alcohol is not a stimulant but a depressant. The apparent stimulant effect is due to early depression of inhibitory areas in the brain. In small amounts, alcohol is a euphoriant. Large amounts cause more and more depression, confusion, disorganization, loss of memory and perception, loss of coordination, and, eventually, loss of consciousness and death.

Alcohol abuse Excessive use of alcohol.

Alcoholic Person suffering from alcoholism. *See* Alcoholism.

Alcoholic seizure *See* Delerium tremens.

Alcoholism Compulsive, frequent drinking of alcohol to the point where it adversely affects the drinker either with respect to health, economically, or socially. Considered medically as a disease characterized by inability to control drinking and resorted to in order to deal with physical or emotional distress.

Alice B. Toklas Brownies Cookies baked with marihuana or hashish. From Alice B. Toklas, female companion and cook for expatriate author Gertrude Stein during the 1920s and 1930s in Paris, who used hashish in a fudge recipe.

Alienation Sense of dissociation from others.

Alkaloid Chemicals containing nitrogen, carbon, oxygen, and hydrogen in plants that may or may not be pharmacologically active.

All Geezed Up Under the influence of narcotics.

All Lit Up Under the influence of a drug; euphoric after drug use.

Alliance for Cannabis Therapeutics (ACT) Alliance of individuals from various aspects of society, e.g., doctors, researchers, politicians, and patients, desirous of ending restrictions against medical use of cannabis.

Alpha Powder Narcotics in powder form.

Alphaprodine Synthetic analog of morphine. Manufactured under the names of Nisentil, Nisintil, and Prisiliden.

Altar Opium pipe.

Altered state of consciousness Psychological state in which perception is altered by drug use.

Amanita muscaria Mushroom which produces hallucinations. Also called fly agaric.

American Council on Marijuana and Other Psychoactive Drugs (ACM) Organization of individuals concerned about the extent of drug abuse, especially marihuana.

Amies Barbiturates.

Amine Molecular compound occurring in many natural and synthetic substances that have biological actions.

Amines, sympathomimetic *See* Sympathomimetic amines.

Amitriptyline Antidepressant drug. Trade name is Elavil.

Amobarbital Intermediate-acting barbiturate classified as sedative/hypnotic. Trade name is Amytal.

Amoeba PCP.

Amorphia California-based lobbying group for legalization of marihuana in the early 1970s.

Amotivational syndrome Sense of apathy, inability to pursue long-term goals, and poor motivation associated with use of marihuana.

Amp 1. Ampule. 2. Amphetamine.

Amped Under the influence of amphetamine.

Amphetamine sulfate Amphetamine compound. Trade name is Benzedrine.

Amphetamines General term for class of drugs that causes stimulation of the brain. These drugs are also called sympathomimetic amines since they are similar in structure and function to endogenous neurotransmitters. There are three types, which vary in potency. Amphetamine sulfate (Benzedrine) is the least potent, methamphetamine hydrochloride (Methedrine, Desoxyn, Amphedroxyn, Norodin) is the most potent, and Dextroamphetamine sulfate (Dexedrine, Dexamyl) has intermediate effects. Usually sold in the form of capsules and tablets but also in powder or liquid form. Most amphetamines in tablet form are amphetamine sulfate, which are sold in the form of small white pills with crosses etched in them. Benzedrine, another form of amphetamine sulfate, comes in the shape of red-colored tablets or football-shaped tablets. Methedrine usually comes in the form of crystals, which are often injected but are also sometimes swallowed or sniffed.

Amphetamines are used as mood elevators, energizers, antidepressants, appetite depressants, and as substances that cause increased alertness and activity. Initial effects are general euphoria, increased talkativeness, and increased concentration. After the effects wear off, a sense of depression may develop, and to counteract this sense the user is likely to take more of the drug. This procedure of taking the drug for sustained periods is called a "run" and may last as long as four or five days during which little or no food is eaten and the user gets very little sleep. Chronic use can result in delusions, hallucinations, paranoia, and psychoses.

The effects of amphetamines are believed to be due to their ability to concentrate biogenic amines in the synapses by blocking their re-uptake and enhancing their release. The general effect resulting from this action is arousal in the peripheral nervous system. Amphetamines cause constriction of blood vessels, increased heart rate, increased blood pressure, and increased muscle tension.

Amps Amphetamines.

Amt Amphetamines.

Amuck, Amok Uncontrollable behavior following drug use, generally involving violence.

Amy 1. Amyl nitrite. 2. Amphetamines.

Amyl nitrite Volatile, clear yellow liquid inhalant generally sold in small fragile glass vial which can easily be crushed between the fingers and then held up to the nose. Has a fruity odor. Classification is stimulant. Causes dilation of small blood vessels and relaxes smooth muscle. Used as an aphrodisiac. Trade name is Aspirol.

Amytal Sodium Trade name for sodium amobarbital. Slang terms, like blue birds, blues, blue heavens, are based on color of the capsule container.

Analeptic Stimulant.

Analgesics Pain reducers. Compounds produce decreased perception of pain (analgesia) without loss of consciousness. The three categories of analgesics are opiate narcotics, nonnarcotic prescription drugs, and nonnarcotic, nonprescription drugs.

Analog Compound similar to another compound in effect but differing somewhat in structure and origin.

Anaphrodisiac A substance that decreases libido.

Anesthetics Pain reducers. Cause lack of sensation. The two types are general anesthetics, which also cause lack of consciousness, and local anesthetics, which cause loss of sensation only in the area to which they are applied.

Angel Someone easily taken advantage of.

Angel Dust 1. PCP. 2. Relatively pure PCP diluted with corn sugar. 3. Parsley sprinkled with PCP. 4. Heroin. 5. Cocaine. 6. Finely chopped marihuana.

Angel Hair PCP.

Angel Mist PCP.

Angel Puke PCP.

Angola Black Potent marihuana from Angola, black in color.

Anileridine Synthetic analog of morphine.

Animal 1. LSD. 2. PCP.

Animal Tranquilizer PCP.

Ann Arbor Ordinance First local law in the United States decriminalizing marihuana use from a felony offense to a misdemeanor with a maximum sentence of 90 days in jail or a $100 fine. Enacted in 1971.

Anodynes *Same as* Analgesics.

Anorectic Drug that causes loss of appetite.

Anslinger, Harry Jacob (1892–1975) Commissioner of the Federal Bureau of Narcotics from 1930 to 1962. The law enforcement official most closely linked with antimarihuana laws in America.

Antabuse Drug used to help alcoholics abstain. Causes an unpleasant reaction when alcohol is consumed.

Antagonist Compound that blocks or counteracts the effects of another compound, the agonist.

Antaphrodisiac *Same as* Anaphrodisiac.

Antidepressants Drugs that elevate mood. They are generally divided into two main types, the tricyclic antidepressants such as amitriptyline hydrochloride (Elavil) and imipramine (Tofranil), and the monoamine oxidase inhibitors such as tranylcypromine (Parnate). These compounds are used for nonmedical purposes only to a minor extent since they have little impact on normal mood and do not produce immediate pleasurable sensations.

Antidote Hypodermic syringe.

Antifreeze 1. Alcohol. 2. Heroin.

Antihistamines Compounds that inhibit the effects of histamine, a naturally occurring substance in the body that causes allergy-related effects such as sneezing. Classified as a nonbarbiturate sedative/hypnotic. Sometimes used in conjunction with alcohol and codeine.

Antiparaphernalia law Law banning the sale of paraphernalia associated with illicit drug use such as marihuana cigarette paper. The first statewide law was passed in Indiana in 1977.

Anxiolytics Sedative/hypnotics.

Anywhere Possessing or smoking marihuana.

Aphrodisiac Substance that increases libido or sexual performance. From Greek goddess of love, Aphrodite.

Apostle Cooked opium pill.

Apple 1. Seconal. 2. Any drug in a red capsule. 3. Non–drug user.

Aprobarbs Barbital.

Arctic Explorer 1. Cocaine user. 2. Narcotics user.

Ardent Spirits Alcohol.

Arecoline Alkaloid found in the betel nut. Has stimulant actions.

Army Disease Addiction to morphine. Term current after Civil War because of large numbers of veterans given morphine to reduce the pain of wounds.

Aroma of Man Brand name for amyl nitrite.

Around the Turn Beyond the maximal pain of withdrawal from narcotics, a state occurring about two to three days after abstinence.

Arsenal 1. Narcotics in a capsule that is concealed in the rectum. Practice resorted to in jail where security is rigid. 2. Hidden supply of narcotics belonging to seller or user.

Artillery Paraphernalia associated with injection of narcotics. Usually a hypodermic needle fitted to a medicine dropper or syringe, a spoon in which to cook the narcotics, and a piece of cotton to filter the drug solution.

Ashes Marihuana.

Ask for Cotton To ask for the cotton just used by another narcotics user so that the residue can be squeezed out and used for a small injection. Person making the request has no money to buy his own.

Aspirol Trade name for amyl nitrite.

Assay Method of determining presence or quantity of a drug in a sample.

Asscache Drugs concealed in a capsule hidden in the rectum.

At Where something related to drug use is taking place.

Ataractic Tranquilizer.

Ataxia Uncoordination.

Atom Bomb Cigarette made of a combination of drugs, for example, marihuana and heroin.

Aunt Hazel Heroin.

Aunt Mary Marihuana.

Aunt Nora Narcotics.

Auntie Opium.

Aurora Borealis PCP.

Autograph Intravenous injection of a narcotic.

Away 1. In jail. 2. No longer using drugs.

Away from the Habit No longer using narcotics.

B

B 1. Drug container. *Same as* Bag, Baggie. 2. Benzedrine.

B.B. Blue Bomber. 10-milligram capsule of Valium.

B Bomb Inhaler for Benzedrine.

Baby 1. Marihuana. 2. Recently begun narcotics habit.

Baby Buds Marihuana.

Babysit To guide someone through a drug-taking experience.

Babysitter Guide who does not take drugs at a party but "controls" and supports those who do if needed.

BAC Blood alcohol concentration.

Back Up To allow blood to re-enter the syringe during intravenous narcotics injection, so that user is sure that the needle is in the vein.

Backed Up Under the influence of narcotics.

Backtrack *Same as* Back Up.

Backwards Barbiturates.

Bad 1. Unpleasant; painful. 2. Good; excellent.

Bad Acid LSD containing impurities that cause unpleasant drug experience.

Bad Bundle Inferior-quality heroin.

Bad Go Very small amount of drug received for money paid.

Bad Head Mentally confused as a result of drug use.

Bad Scene Unpleasant situation.

Bad Seed Mescaline.

Bad Trip Unpleasant drug reaction, for example, panic and anxiety. Generally associated with LSD, but also with other drugs.

Bag, Baggie Plastic sandwich bag containing about 1 ounce of marihuana, or small glassine bag containing a quantity of heroin (about 5 milligrams, to which milk sugar or quinine has been added).

Bag Lady Female narcotics seller.

Bag Man Narcotics seller.

Baking Soda Base Cocaine freebase made with baking soda rather than flammable solvents.

Bala Seconal.

Bale Kilogram or pound of drugs.

Bale of Hay Unspecified amount of marihuana, usually 1 kilogram or pound.

Balloon Room Place where marihuana is smoked.

Balloon Room without a Parachute Place where no marihuana is left.

Balloons Drugs sold in balloons. Can be swallowed to avoid detection.

Balot Heroin.

Bam 1. Amphetamines. 2. Combination of amphetamines and barbiturates.

Bambalacha Marihuana, hashish.

Bambalacha Rambler Marihuana smoker.

Bambita Amphetamine.

Bamboo Opium pipe.

Bamboo Puffer Opium smoker.

Bambu Brand of marihuana cigarette paper. Most popular brand among the beatniks of the 1950s.

Bambu case Metal container for marihuana cigarette paper.

Bammy, Bammies, Bams Low-potency marihuana cigarettes.

Bams Amphetamines.

Ban Apple Brand name for amyl nitrite.

Banana Cigarette paper used to make marihuana cigarettes.

Banana smoking *See* Mellow Yellow.

Banana Splits Amyl nitrite ampules.

Banana with Cheese Marihuana cigarette to which cocaine freebase has been added.

Banewort Belladonna.

Bang 1. Narcotics. 2. Injection of narcotics. 3. Marihuana. 4. To smoke marihuana.

Bang in the Arm Intravenous injection of narcotics.

Bang Room Place where narcotics are used.

Bangster Narcotics user who injects drug intravenously.

Bangue *See* Bhang.

Bank Bandits Barbiturates.

Bar Compressed block of marihuana stuck together with sugar, honey, or Coca-Cola.

Barbital Long-acting barbiturate. First introduced into medical practice in 1903 under the trade name of Veronal. Comes in the form of white powder, tablets, and capsules.

Barbiturates Class of drugs that cause depression of the central nervous system. Usually they are taken to reduce anxiety or to induce euphoria.

First manufactured around 1850. Presently over 2,500 variants have been synthesized, but only about 15 are used in medical practice. The most popular varieties subject to abuse are Amytal, Nembutal, Seconal, and Tuinal. These are considered to be short- and intermediate-acting in effect. The drugs come in the form of capsules of various colors or tablets. In most cases barbiturates are taken by mouth, but they can also be taken by intravenous injection.

Small doses produce a calming effect. However, some users do become hostile and violent following ingestion. As the dosage is increased, effects progress through sedation, sleep, coma, and death. Prolonged use can result in dependence. Withdrawal can be more dangerous than withdrawal from narcotics and can involve anxiety, loss of appetite, insomnia, muscle twitching, convulsions, and psychoses. Overdosing, especially when barbiturates are taken in conjunction with alcohol, accounts annually for several thousand deaths.

Barbs Barbiturates.

Barmecide Morphine.

Barrel LSD.

Base Cocaine freebase.

Base Binge Long period of continual use of cocaine freebase without intervening sleep.

Base Dreams Dreams concerning purchase, preparation, or use of cocaine.

Baseball Smoking cocaine freebase.

Baseman Cocaine freebase smoker. *See* First Baseman; Second Baseman.

Bash 1. Good time; a party. 2. Marihuana.

Basted Intoxicated by a drug.

Bay State Hypodermic needle.

Bayonet Hypodermic needle.

B-bomb Benzedrine inhaler.

BBs Burnout as a result of chronic and extensive use of cocaine freebase.

Be in Business To be dependent on narcotics.

Be in Tweeds To smoke marihuana.

Be On To be dependent on narcotics.

Be Sent To be satisfied and in a stupor from smoking marihuana.

Be Up Against It To use narcotics.

Be Washed Up To undergo withdrawal from narcotics.

Beam Test Forensic test for detecting presence of marihuana in an unknown material.

Beaming Intoxicated by a drug.

Bean 1. Benzedrine. 2. Mescaline. 3. Amphetamine.

Bean Head Chronic user of Benzedrine.

Bean Trip Experience due to use of Benzedrine.

Beans 1. Peyote. 2. Amphetamines.

Beast LSD.

Beat To cheat someone out of his money.

Beat Pad Place where low-potency marihuana is sold.

Beat the Gong To smoke opium.

Beat the Weeds To smoke marihuana.

Beaten Unable to function normally as a result of chronic drug use.

Beautiful Lady Belladonna.

Bed Bugs Companion narcotics users.

Bee *See* Bag, Baggie.

Bee That Stings Drug dependence.

Behind Using a drug, for example, *behind acid* means "using LSD."

Belladonna 1. Drugs originating from the deadly nightshade plant, for example, strammonium, hyocyanamine. Main active ingredients are atropine and scopolamine. Sometimes added to LSD to intensify effects. 2. PCP.

Belly Habit Using narcotics. From the stomach cramps associated with withdrawal from narcotics.

Belt 1. Drink of alcohol or injection of drug. 2. Euphoria following drug use.

Belt Padding Drug tolerance—the need to increase the amount of drug taken in order to experience the same sensations as experienced when the drug was first taken.

Belted Intoxicated.

Bend the Habit To reduce the amount of drug so as to become less dependent.

Bend the Needle To try to become less drug-dependent without success.

Bender Prolonged period of alcohol or drug consumption.

Bending Under the influence of a drug.

Bending and Bowing *Same as* Bending.

Bending the Head Smoking marihuana.

Benny Benzedrine.

Benny Jag Benzedrine intoxication.

Bent Under the influence of a drug.

Bent Out of Shape 1. Angry, disgruntled. 2. Intoxicated by a drug.

Benz Benzedrine.

Benzadrina Homosexual who uses amphetamines regularly.

Benzedrine Trade name for amphetamine sulfate. Sold in the form of heart-shaped tablets and, at higher doses, red and clear capsules.

Benzodiazepine Class of drugs to which Valium and Librium belong. Classified as nonhypnotic sedatives and muscle relaxants.

Bernice, Bernies Cocaine. Possibly derived from an early patent medicine used to treat colds which contained cocaine.

Bernie's Flake Cocaine.

Bethesda Gold Marihuana, not very potent.

Betting on the Horse Dependence on heroin.

Bhang Marihuana. One of the oldest terms used in reference to the dried leaves of the cannabis plant. In India, a beverage made with marihuana. Term is believed to be derived from the Sanskrit *bhanga*.

Bible Physicians' Desk Reference. *See* Book.

Big Bag Ten-dollar bag of heroin.

Big Bloke Cocaine.

Big Boy Heroin.

Big C Cocaine.

Big Chief Mescaline.

Big D 1. LSD. 2. Dilaudid.

Big H Heroin.

Big Harry Heroin.

Big John Police officer.

Big M Morphine.

Big Man Drug dealer who supplies the pusher.

Big O Opium.

Big Shot Connection Middleman in distribution of drugs between street sellers and importers.

Billie Hoak Cocaine.

Billied Dependent on cocaine.

Bim Police officer.

Bindle Small amount of narcotics wrapped in cellophane.

Bindle Kate Female narcotics user.

Bindle Stiff Narcotics user.

Bindle Stiffened Dependent on narcotics.

Bing 1. Injection of narcotics. 2. Small amount of narcotics.

Bing Room Place where narcotics are taken.

Binge Short, intense period of alcohol or drug use.

Bingle 1. Narcotics. 2. Drug seller.

Bingo Amount of narcotics to be injected.

Bingo Room Place where narcotics are used.

Biphetamine Drug containing combination of amphetamines.

Birdcage Place where a Birdcage Hype sleeps.

Birdcage Hype Destitute narcotics user.

Birdhouse Run-down hotel where narcotics are sold.

Birdhouse Hype Narcotics user who buys drugs in a Birdhouse.

Birdie Powder 1. Cocaine. 2. Morphine.

Birdie Stuff Narcotics.

Bird's Eye Small amount of narcotics.

Birdwood Marihuana.

Biscuits Methadone.

Bit 1. Personal interests. 2. Time spent in jail.

Bite Dependence on narcotics.

Bite One's Lip To smoke marihuana.

Bitten by White Mosquitoes Using cocaine.

Biz, Bizz Paraphernalia for intravenous injection. *Same as* Artillery.

Black 1. Opium. 2. Potent hashish. Usually kept by dealers for their own use.

Black and White Police car.

Black Beauties 1. Amphetamines or barbiturates. 2. Biphetamine capsules.

Black Birds Amphetamines.

Black Bombers Amphetamines.

Black Bottle 1. Narcotics. 2. Chloral hydrate.

Black Columbus Marihuana.

Black Gold Potent marihuana.

Black Gungeon, Gunion Potent marihuana, viscous and black. Derived from the Jamaican term *ganja*, which in turn originated from the Indian term *ganga*.

Black Hash Hashish.

Black Jack 1. Paregoric which has been heated to concentrate it for intravenous injection. 2. Brand name for amyl nitrite.

Black Mo, Moat, Mold, Monte, Mota Potent marihuana. Marihuana mixed with sugar or honey. Popular in the 1940s as *muta*, a Mexican term for marihuana.

Black Mollies Barbiturates.

Black Oil Hashish oil. Dark black in appearance. Appeared around 1972 in California.

Black Out Period of amnesia following heavy consumption of alcohol.

Black Pills Opium.

Black Russian Hashish from Russia.

Black Shit Opium.

Black Smoke Opium.

Black Spot Place where opium is smoked.

Black Stuff 1. Opium that is made ready for smoking. 2. Dark brown heroin.

Black Tabs LSD.

Black Whack PCP.

Black Widow Capsule containing amphetamines and barbiturates.

Blanco Heroin.

Blanco y Negro Brand of marihuana cigarette papers, literally "black and white."

Blank 1. Low-potency marihuana. 2. Quantity of alleged drug found to contain only inert material.

Blanket Papers for making marihuana cigarettes.

Blast 1. Rapid, strong effect from using a drug. 2. To smoke marihuana.

Blast a Joint, Reefers, Stick, Weed To smoke marihuana.

Blast Mary Jane To smoke marihuana.

Blast Party Party where marihuana is smoked.

Blast Reefers To smoke marihuana.

Blast Weed To smoke marihuana.

Blasted Under the influence of marihuana.

Blind Very intoxicated by a drug.

Blind Munchies Overwhelming craving for any kind of food after smoking marihuana.

Blinky Cocaine freebase.

Blitzed Very intoxicated by a drug.

Block 1. One kilogram (2.2 pounds) of marihuana. 2. Small amount of narcotics, less than 1 ounce.

Blockbusters Barbiturates.

Blocked Under the influence of marihuana.

Bloker Chronic user of cocaine.

Blond Hashish from Lebanon or Morocco, light yellow in color.

Blotter 1. Absorbent paper on which LSD solution has been placed. 2. Residue of narcotics strained out when solution is passed through cotton.

Blow 1. Cocaine. 2. To smoke marihuana or snort heroin or cocaine.

Blow a Pill To smoke opium.

Blow a Shot To waste a drug because the equipment used to administer it breaks or because of faulty injection.

Blow a Stick To smoke a marihuana cigarette.

Blow a Vein To collapse a vein as a result of frequent intravenous injection into it.

Blow Charlie To sniff cocaine.

Blow Coke To sniff cocaine.

Blow Horse To sniff heroin.

Blow One's Cool 1. To lose self-control. 2. To become angry.

Blow One's Mind 1. To become intoxicated by a drug. 2. To alter consciousness. 3. To lose one's sanity.

Blow One's Top 1. To become intoxicated by marihuana. 2. To become angry.

Blow Snow To sniff cocaine.

Blow the Meet To fail to meet a drug contact at the appointed time.

Blower 1. Marihuana user. 2. Informer.

Blowtop Marihuana user.

Blue Acid LSD.

Blue Angel Capsule of Amytal Sodium.

Blue Birds Capsules of Amytal Sodium.

Blue Bomber 10-milligram capsule of Valium. Color of capsule is blue.

Blue Bullets Capsules of Amytal Sodium.

Blue Chairs LSD.

Blue Cheers LSD.

Blue Cheese Hashish.

Blue Clouds Amobarbital.

Blue de Hue Marihuana. Term used by American soldiers in Vietnam.

Blue Devils Capsules of Amytal Sodium.

Blue Dolls Capsules of Amytal Sodium.

Blue Dot LSD solution on paper.

Blue Fascist Police officer.

Blue Flag LSD.

Blue Funk Deep depression.

Blue Heavens 1. Capsules of Amytal Sodium. 2. LSD.

Blue Jackets Capsules of Amytal Sodium.

Blue Mist LSD.

Blue Morning Morning-glory seeds.

Blue People Syndrome Peripheral cyanosis resulting from using too much cocaine. Characterized by blue color in fingers and toes, probably due to decreased blood supply to these areas.

Blue Sage Marihuana.

Blue Sky Blond Potent marihuana from Colombia.

Blue Splash LSD solution on paper.

Blue Star Morning-glory seeds.

Blue Tips Capsules of Amytal Sodium.

Blue Velvet 1. Amytal Sodium. 2. Combination of paregoric and an antihistamine.

Blue Vials LSD.

Blues 1. Capsules of Amytal Sodium. 2. Barbiturates.

Blunt 1. Barbiturate. 2. Specifically, the barbiturate Seconal.

BNDD *See* Bureau of Narcotics and Dangerous Drugs.

Bo Marihuana from Colombia.

Bo Bo Bush Marihuana.

Bo Bo Jockey Marihuana user.

Body Drugs Drugs that cause physical dependence.

Body Packing To swallow condoms containing drugs in order to smuggle them across borders.

Bogart a Joint To salivate on or be slow to share a marihuana cigarette. Derived from dangling cigarette associated with Humphrey Bogart.

Boggs Act Law enacted in 1951 increasing severity of penalties for violation of drug laws.

Boil Out Cure Attempt to break narcotics dependence by abrupt abstinence in contrast to slower, drug-treated withdrawal.

Bolsa Heroin.

Bolt Brand name for amyl nitrite.

Bolus Small ball of opium.

Bomb, Bomber 1. Thick marihuana cigarette. 2. Heroin.

Bombed Under the influence of marihuana or alcohol; very intoxicated.

Bombida Benzedrine.

Bombido Benzedrine.

Bombita 1. Benzedrine. 2. Combination of amphetamine, barbiturate, and heroin.

Bonaroo 1. Narcotics that have been highly diluted with inert material.

Bong Pipe in which smoker draws from stem attached to upper part of bowl. The bowl fills with smoke and provides a sustained, concentrated flow of smoke allowing smoker to inhale large amounts of smoke and thereby produce a more intense effect. Popular device in Asia. Introduced to America by GIs returning from Vietnam around 1970.

Bonita Heroin.

Boo, Bu Marihuana.

Boo Hoo Priest in Neo-American Church who uses drugs as a religious sacrament.

Boo Reefer Marihuana cigarette.

Boo-gee Thin paper packing between a needle and a medicine dropper used to administer narcotics intravenously.

Book *Physicians' Desk Reference (P.D.R.)*. Standard medical text describing various drugs and their effects.

Booking with Charlie Dependent on morphine.

Boost To shoplift.

Booster Stick Tobacco cigarette to which THC has been added.

Boot 1. Kicks; thrills; excitement. 2. To slowly inject heroin intravenously so that after a little is injected, it is allowed to flow back into the syringe along with some blood, and then another small amount is injected. This is done to prolong the effect of the drug.

Bootlegs Counterfeit drugs.

Boots and Shoes Destitute; having sold shoes for drugs.

Bopper *See* Teenybopper.

Boreroom Beater Marihuana smoker.

Boss Very good; excellent.

Boss Habit High degree of tolerance to narcotics such that a large amount of drug is needed to prevent withdrawal-like symptoms.

Bottle Large container of pills.

Bottles Amphetamines.

Bottom Out To experience the worst possible drug-related condition before emerging and improving.

Bounce Powder Cocaine.

Bounce the Goof Balls To smoke marihuana.

Bouncing Powder Cocaine.

Bow Sow Narcotics.

Bowin Narcotics user.

Box Quantity of marihuana that could fit into a penny matchbox.

Box of L Box of methedrine capsules.

Boxed Intoxicated.

Boy Heroin or marihuana. In contrast to *girl*, the term for cocaine.

Bozo Heroin.

Brain Burned 1. Very intoxicated by a drug. 2. Unable to function normally as a result of chronic drug use.

Brain Ticklers Amphetamines or barbiturates.

Bread Money.

Break a Stick To smoke marihuana.

Break the Habit To no longer be dependent on narcotics.

Break the Needle To try to stop using narcotics.

Breaking In Starting to use narcotics.

Breckenridge Green Low-potency marihuana from Kentucky.

Brew with Hocks Opium.

Brewery 1. Place where drugs are manufactured. 2. Place where opium is smoked.

Brick 1. Kilogram of marihuana compressed into the shape of a brick. 2. Crude opium.

Brick Gum Opium shaped into bricks or cakes.

Bridge Device used to hold a burning marihuana cigarette butt.

Brifo Marihuana. *Variation of* Greefa, Greefo, Grefa, Grifa, Griffa, Grifo.

Bring Down 1. To calm someone who has become agitated from drug use. 2. To return someone to a nonintoxicated state.

Bring Up 1. *Same as* second definition of Boot. 2. To squeeze a vein so that it becomes more prominent, making injection into it easier.

Brink To buy narcotics.

Brisket Small amount of narcotics.

Broach To inject narcotics intravenously.

Broad Shoulders Social worker.

Broccoli Marihuana.

Brody To feign withdrawal in hopes of convincing a physician to administer or prescribe narcotics.

Broker Narcotics seller.

Brother Heroin.

Brown Heroin from Mexico.

Brown Dots LSD.

Brown Rine Heroin.

Brown Rock Heroin crystals.

Brown Shoes Non–drug user.

Brown Stuff Opium.

Brown Sugar Heroin.

Brownies Brown-tipped capsules of amphetamines.

Browns Amphetamines.

Brush Narcotics injection.

Brute Brown coca paste from Colombia.

Bu *Same as* Boo.

Budda, Buddha Sticks Marihuana.

Buffoteine Drug isolated from mushroom (*Amanita muscaria*) related chemically to DMT.

Bug To feign withdrawal in hopes of convincing a physician to administer or prescribe narcotics.

Bug Juice Narcotics.

Bugged Initiated into the use of drugs.

Building a Habit Acquiring drug tolerance.

Bull Police officer.

Bull Horror Paranoia concerning arrest. Individual thinks everyone is a police officer and is disturbed by the slightest sound.

Bull Jive Marihuana adulterated with oregano, catnip, or other impotent material.

Bullet 1. One-year jail sentence. 2. Brand name for amyl nitrite.

Bullet Thai Marihuana from Thailand.

Bum Bend Unpleasant drug experience.

Bum Rap Arrested or convicted when innocent.

Bum Steer Someone who smuggles drugs into prison.

Bum Trip Unpleasant experience from drug use such as anxiety, panic, paranoia.

Bumble Bees Amphetamines.

Bummer 1. Any unpleasant experience. 2. Sense of depression or paranoia from drug use.

Bundle 1. Twenty-five five-dollar bags of heroin, usually held together by a rubber band. 2. The amount purchased by a pusher for resale to the user.

Bunk Opium.

Bunk Fee Admission price to an opium den.

Bunk Habit 1. Opium dependence. 2. Slight dependence on narcotics.

Bunk Yen Opium habit caused by passive inhalation of opium smoke.

Bureau of Narcotics and Dangerous Drugs (BNDD) Federal agency in charge of controlling illicit drugs. Replaced the Federal Bureau of Narcotics in 1968.

Burese Cocaine.

Burn To cheat.

Burn an Indian To smoke marihuana or become dependent on it.

Burn Artist Dishonest drug seller.

Burn Indian Hay To smoke marihuana.

Burn Out 1. To experience mental deterioration from chronic drug use. 2. Someone unable to function normally as a result of chronic drug use.

Burn Test Street test for determining presence of purity of cocaine. Small amount of suspected substance is placed on aluminum foil and heated. Absence of residue indicates complete purity.

Burn the Hay To smoke marihuana.

Burn the Midnight Oil To smoke opium.

Burned 1. Cheated by buying a phony drug, adulterated marihuana, or by not receiving the drug for payment. 2. Recognized; undercover officer's identity exposed.

Burned Out 1. Unable to function normally as a result of prolonged drug use. 2. Giving up drug use.

Burnese Cocaine.

Burnies 1. Marihuana cigarettes. 2. Partially smoked marihuana cigarettes.

Bush Marihuana.

Bush Tea Tea made with marihuana.

Bushwacker Marihuana smoker.

Business 1. *Same as* Biz. 2. Opium den.

Businessman's Lunch, Businessman's Special, Businessman's Trip 1. Amphetamines. 2. DMT.

Businessman's Psychedelic Martini Dimethyltryptamine, a short-acting hallucinogen similar to psilocin.

Businessman's Trip *Same as* Businessman's Psychedelic Martini.

Bust 1. To arrest. 2. An arrest. 3. To smoke marihuana.

Bust a Cap To break a capsule containing narcotics.

Bust the Mainline To inject narcotics intravenously.

Busted Arrested.

Buster Federal narcotics officer.

Busters Barbiturates.

Busy Bee PCP.

Butt Marihuana cigarette.

Butter Flower Marihuana.

Button 1. Peyote. 2. Small bolus of opium.

Butyl nitrite Drug similar to amyl nitrite.

Buy To purchase marihuana.

Buzz 1. Early sensations as the effects of a drug begin to be felt. 2. Mild euphoric feeling from smoking marihuana. 3. Intoxicated.

Buzzed Slightly intoxicated by marihuana or alcohol.

Buzzing Trying to make a drug purchase.

BZ STP.

C

C Cocaine.

C and H Mixture of cocaine and heroin.

C and M Mixture of cocaine and morphine.

Caballo Heroin; Spanish slang for the drug.

Cabello Cocaine.

Ca-ca Heroin.

Cache Hiding place for drugs. *Same as* Stache.

Cacil Cocaine.

Cactus Mescaline.

Cactus Button Mescaline.

Cadet Naive drug user.

Cadillac 1. Cocaine. 2. PCP. 3. High-quality drugs.

Caffeine Ingredient found in coffee, tea, cocoa, and various soft drinks. Stimulates the central nervous system.

Caffeinism Dependence on caffeine.

Caines Local anesthetics, e.g., lidocaine, used to adulterate cocaine.

California Poppy State flower of California. Does not contain opiates, but does contain some of the other materials in opium. Does not produce dependence.

California Sunshine LSD.

Call Sense of exhilaration following injection of narcotics.

Cam Red Cambodian Red. Potent marihuana from Cambodia.

Came Cocaine.

Campfire Boy Opium user.

Camphor Material sometimes mixed with marihuana. Produces slight exhilaration.

Can Ounce of marihuana.

Canadian Black Marihuana grown in Canada.

Canadian Bouncer Seconal from Canada.

Canadian Quail Methaqualone.

Canal Vein into which narcotics are injected.

Canary Nembutal, a barbiturate.

Cancelled Stick Tobacco cigarette from which tobacco has been removed and replaced with marihuana.

Candied Dependent on cocaine.

Candy 1. Cocaine. 2. LSD. 3. Hashish. 4. Barbiturates.

Candy a J(oint) To add another potent drug, for example, heroin, to a marihuana cigarette.

Candy Bar Cocaine seller.

Candy Cee Cocaine.

Candy Fiend Chronic and heavy user of cocaine.

Candy Head *Same as* Candy Fiend.

Candy Man Drug seller.

Cannabidiol (CBD) Cannabinoid occurring in marihuana. Does not possess psychoactive properties.

Cannabinism Psychosis resulting from marihuana usage.

Cannabinol 1. Cannabinoid occurring in marihuana. 2. Misnomer for PCP.

Cannabis Herb from which marihuana, hashish, and the like are obtained. Cannabis is a member of the Cannabicae family which includes *Cannabis sativa, Cannabis indica,* and *Cannabis ruderalis.* Cannabis is one of the oldest plants cultivated by man. Its leaves and flowering tops are used for their psychoactive ingredient, delta–9-THC; the stem is the source of fiber known as hemp, used to make rope, twine, cloth, and many other products; and the seeds have been used as food for both men and birds. The oil within the seeds has also been used as a base for paints.

The psychoactive potency of marihuana depends on the concentration of delta–9-THC produced by the plant and is determined by genetic and climatic factors.

Cannabis grown for its fiber contains very little THC (less than 0.5 percent) but has a high cannabidiol (CBD) content, whereas that grown for its psychoactive effects may contain upward of 20 percent THC and very little CBD.

Cannabis indica Marihuana plant originating in India, literally "Indian cane." *Cannabis indica* was identified in 1783 by French naturalist Lamarck as being distinct from *Cannabis sativa* because of *sativa*'s woodier stem, shorter height (about 4 feet), denser branching, and the greater strength of its psychoactive properties.

Cannabis ruderalis Species of cannabis occurring in wild state in Central Asia. Differs from *C. indica* and *C. sativa* in being much smaller (up to 2 feet), having fewer branches, shorter leaves, and smaller seeds.

Cannabis sativa Literally "cultivated cane." This botanical name was proposed in 1753 by Swedish botanist Carolus Linnaeus. The term is derived from *cana* (Sanskrit, "cane" or "reed") *bios* (Greek, " bow") and *sativa* (Latin, "cultivated").

Canned Goods Any drug. Term derived from the selling of drugs such as marihuana in Prince Albert tobacco cans in the 1930s.

Canned Stuff *Same as* Canned Goods.

Cannon Hypodermic syringe.

Cannon Ball Mixture of heroin and cocaine.

Cap 1. To purchase drugs. 2. To open a drug capsule containing narcotics so that the drug inside can be dissolved for intravenous injection. 3. Drug capsule containing narcotics. 4. Any drug capsule.

Cap Out To become drowsy or sleepy from taking marihuana.

Capping To put drugs into capsules.

Carbona Cleaning fluid inhalant.

Carboxylation Chemical conversion of inactive cannabinoid acids into active substances when heated.

Carburetor Tube with one or more holes in its side. A cigarette is placed in one end and inhaled through the other with the holes on the side covered. When the tube is filled, the holes on the side are uncovered; this causes smoke to be drawn forcefully into the lungs. *Same as* Shotgun.

Card Small amount of narcotics. Derived from the amount of opium sold by Chinese dealers after it had been weighed on the back of a playing card.

Career Life-style relating to the procurement and use of heroin, for example, stealing to obtain money to buy it, usage, treatment for withdrawal, avoiding detection.

Cargo Supply of drugs for sale.

Carmabus Marihuana.

Caronotics Narcotics.

Carrie Cocaine.

Carrie Nation Cocaine.

Carry 1. Period prior to feelings of withdrawal. 2. To have drugs in one's possession.

Carrying Possessing drugs.

Cartwheel To feign withdrawal in hopes of convincing a physician to administer or prescribe narcotics.

Cartwheels Amphetamines. Derived from the X-shaped score on tablets.

Case Study Detailed information about an individual and/or his or her family relating to use of drugs or any other psychosocial or medical consideration.

Cash a Script To have a counterfeit prescription filled.

Casing the Nurse Dependent on narcotics.

Cat Member of an "in-group."

Cat Nap Short period of sleep during withdrawal.

Catch Up To undergo withdrawal from narcotics.

Catecholamines Group of biochemicals with a similar structure produced in the adrenal glands and in nerve endings, for example, norepinephrine, dopamine, epinephrine. Many drugs are believed to produce their psychoactive effects by being similar in structure to these compounds.

Catholic Aspirin Amphetamines. Derived from shape of cross on tablets.

Catnip Herb sometimes mixed with marihuana to increase its bulk so that more money can be charged. Sometimes catnip alone is sold as marihuana to naive buyers.

Cat's Meow Brand name for amyl nitrite.

Cat-tail Marihuana cigarette.

Caught in a Snow Storm Intoxicated by cocaine.

Caught on the Needle Dependent on narcotics.

Cave Abscess due to collapse of vein at site of narcotics injection.

Cave Digging Looking for an area in a collapsed vein where an injection can still be made.

CB Doriden. From the name of the manufacturer, Ciba.

C-duct Cocaine.

Cecil 1. Cocaine. 2. Narcotics.

Cecil Jones Someone dependent on narcotics.

Ceciled Dependent on narcotics.

Cee Cocaine.

Cement Narcotics sold at wholesale.

Cent One doller.

Center for Multicultural Awareness Part of the National Institute on Drug Abuse. Involved in drug abuse prevention programs for minorities.

Central nervous system The brain and spinal cord.

Chalk 1. Cocaine. 2. Amphetamines. 3. Methadone.

Chalked Up Intoxicated by cocaine.

Champ Drug user who does not inform on his supplier or other drug users.

Chandoo, Chandu Opium prepared for smoking.

Channel 1. Vein into which narcotics are injected. 2. Narcotics user who injects drugs intravenously.

Channel Line Vein into which narcotics are injected.

Channel Swimmer Narcotics user who injects drug intravenously.

Charas Hashish. Term is Indian in origin and is still used in India to refer to high-potency cannabis.

Charge 1. Marihuana. 2. Intoxicated by a drug. 3. Originally, the reaction to narcotics.

Charged Up Under the influence of narcotics.

Charley, Charlie 1. Cocaine. 2. Cocaine user.

Charley Coke Cocaine user.

Charley Cotton Cotton used to strain impurities from solution of narcotics prior to intravenous injection.

Charras Marihuana.

Chasing the Bag Trying to get the best-quality heroin available for the day.

Chasing the Dragon Heating heroin so that the fumes can be inhaled. As the drug is heated, it takes the form of a snake or dragon and is inhaled through a paper tube.

Chasing the Nurse Dependent on morphine.

Chasing the White Nurse Dependent on morphine.

C-Head Chronic cocaine user.

Cheating Using illicit drugs while in a drug treatment program.

Check Small amount of narcotics.

Cheeo Marihuana seeds.

Cheese Cocaine freebase.

Chef 1. To prepare opium for smoking by rolling it into pills or warming the pipe. 2. Individual who prepares opium. 3. Individual who prepares cocaine freebase.

Cherry Leb Hashish oil.

Cherry Top LSD.

Chew the Fat Dependent on narcotics.

Chewing the Gum Dependent on opium.

Chiba Chiba Marihuana.

Chicago Black Potent marihuana, black in color.

Chicago Green Potent marihuana, green in color.

Chicago Leprosy Abscesses throughout the body from frequent injection.

Chicharra Mixture of marihuana and tobacco.

Chick Cocaine.

Chicken Powder Amphetamine powder.

Chicken Shit Habit Use of small amount of drugs.

Chicory Poor-quality opium. Probably derived from analogy with the use of chicory as a coffee substitute during World War II.

Chief, the LSD.

Chill To refuse to sell drugs to a prospective buyer.

Chillum Cone-shaped pipe for smoking marihuana. Marihuana is packed into the top part of the cone. The bottom of the cone is covered with a cloth, held in the hand, and smoke is inhaled from cupped hands.

China White 1. Heroin. 2. Derivative of Demerol; narcoticlike drug with much higher potency than morphine. Also called synthetic heroin.

Chinaman 1. Dependent on narcotics. 2. Experiencing withdrawal from narcotics.

Chinaman on (One's) Back Dependence on narcotics. A very old expression derived from the association of opium use and the Chinese in San Francisco during the turn of the century.

Chinaman's Distress Withdrawal from narcotics.

Chinese Molasses Opium.

Chinese Needle Work Intravenous narcotics injection.

Chinese Red Heroin.

Chinese Saxophone Opium pipe.

Chinese White High-potency heroin.

Chip 1. Irregular use of narcotics. 2. To dilute narcotics with inert material.

Chipper Occasional narcotics user.

Chipping Occasional narcotics use.

Chippy *Same as* Chipper.

Chippy Habit *Same as* Chip.

Chira Marihuana. Term is derived from Charas.

Chiva Heroin.

Chloral hydrate Trichloroacetaldehyde. Sedative/hypnotic drug first synthesized in 1862. The oldest of the hypnotic (sleep-inducing) drugs. Use decreased after introduction of barbiturates, but is still widely used. Sold in the form of syrups and soft gelatin capsules. Has slightly acrid smell and bitter caustic taste. Chronic use can result in tolerance and dependence. Withdrawal resembles delirium tremens. When combined with alcohol it produces rapid intoxication. Combination was known as a Mickey Finn or Knockout Drops.

Chlordiazepoxide Librium. Antianxiety drug belonging to the benzodiazepine group of drugs that also includes Valium.

Chlorodyne Stomach remedy that contained marihuana, manufactured by Squibb Company in the late nineteenth and early twentieth centuries.

Chloroform Vaporous anesthetic that can produce intoxicationlike effects when inhaled in small amounts.

Chlorpromazine Antipsychotic tranquilizer. Trade name is Thorazine.

Chocolate 1. Hashish. 2. Opium.

Chocolate Chips LSD.

Choker Regular cigarette to which cocaine has been added.

Cholly, Cholley Cocaine.

Christian Methamphetamine. *See* Catholic Aspirin.

Christina Methamphetamine.

Christmas Roll Collection of barbiturate capsules. Term derives from the many colors of the capsules.

Christmas Tree Capsule containing amphetamines and barbiturates.

Chromatography Chemical method for detecting and identifying drugs present in unknown substances containing them. Substances are absorbed on a paper or column containing a solvent. Identity is determined by comparing movement with a known material.

Chronic 1. Long-term; opposite of acute. 2. Narcotics user.

Chuck a Wingding To feign withdrawal in hopes of convincing a physician to administer or prescribe narcotics.

Chuck Habit, Chuckers Overwhelming desire for food following withdrawal from narcotics.

Chuck Horrors Disgust for food experienced during withdrawal from narcotics.

Chuckers, Chucks Appetite, craving, hunger for food after smoking marihuana.

Chunk Hashish.

Churus Marihuana. Term is derived from Charas.

Cibas Doriden, nonbarbiturate sedative/hypnotic made by Ciba Company.

Cigar Thick marihuana cigarette.

Cigarrode Cristal PCP.

Circus *Same as* Chuck a Wingding.

Citroli Potent hashish from Nepal.

CJ 1. PCP. 2. Crystal Joint.

C-jam Cocaine.

Clarabelle THC—Tetrahydrocannabinol, the psychoactive ingredient in marihuana.

Clay THC—Tetrahydrocannabinol, the psychoactive ingredient in marihuana.

Clean 1. To remove stems and seeds from crude marihuana. 2. Not using drugs. 3. Not having drugs in one's possession.

Clean Up To stop using drugs.

Cleaned No longer dependent on drugs.

Clear Up To stop using drugs.

Clearlight LSD solution on paper.

Client Oriented Data Acquisition Process (CODAP) Federal program reporting drugs used by patients in federal drug abuse treatment programs.

Clime's on you Intoxicated by a drug. Expression used during the 1930s and 1940s.

Clip 1. Device used to hold a burning marihuana cigarette butt. 2. To arrest.

Clipped Arrested.

Clordiazepoxide Chemical name for Librium, an antianxiety tranquilizer.

Clorox Test Street test for determining purity of cocaine and possible presence of adulterants. Substance is added to glass containing Clorox bleach. Pure cocaine spreads out in streams; adulterants such as lidocaine remain on surface.

Cloud Nine Under the influence of a drug.

Clown To feign withdrawal in hopes of convincing a physician to administer or prescribe narcotics.

Club Place where marihuana is smoked. Term was used in the 1930s, when such places existed somewhat analogously to a bar.

Club des Haschischins A social club of French writers and artists who met on a monthly basis in Paris's Latin Quarter during the 1830s and 1840s to fraternize and use hashish. Founded by Theophile Gautier, the club included such notables as Alexander Dumas, Victor Hugo, Charles Baudelaire, Gerard de Nerval, and Ferdinand Boissard.

CNS Central nervous system.

Coast *See* Coasting.

Coasting 1. Feeling euphoric following drug use. 2. Under the influence of a drug.

Coast-to-coasts Long-lasting amphetamines. From the use of amphetamines by long-distance truck drivers.

Cobalt test Field-testing method to determine if cocaine is present. Cocaine is added to solution of cobalt thiocyanate. If solution turns immediately blue, cocaine is present in a relatively high concentration. Appearance of dark blue flecks followed by blue color indicates less-potent cocaine. Procaine will also cause blue color to form.

Cobics Heroin.

Cobies Morphine.

Coby *Same as* Cobies.

Coca 1. Plant (*Erythroxylon coca*) from which cocaine is derived. Coca is native to the mountains of South and Central America. 2. Cocaine.

Coca Paste Crude extract of coca.

Cocaine Primary psychoactive ingredient in coca. Cocaine was isolated from coca (*Erythroxylon coca*) in the 1850s. Initially it was used as a local anesthetic in eye surgery. Also used in nose and throat surgery because it constricts blood vessels and thereby reduces bleeding. Sold in the form of white crystals, called flake, or powder that is sometimes diluted to about half its volume by lactose or other inert material. Drug is often "snorted" through the nose, but it is also sometimes injected intravenously.

Pharmacologically, cocaine resembles the amphetamines in its stimulant actions. In 1914 it was included in the Harrison Narcotics Act list of narcotic drugs. It is now included under Schedule 2 of controlled Substances Act. Effects include euphoria, elation, arousal, accelerated thought processes, increased sense of confidence. Negative reactions include hand tremor, nausea, sweating, insomnia, increased blood pressure and pulse, paranoia involving fear of police detection, apathy, and confusion. Chronic use of high doses has been associated with psychosis involving depression and hallucination.

Cocaine Anonymous Self-help group for cocaine users, patterned on Alcoholics Anonymous.

Cocaine Blues Depression associated with frequent use of cocaine.

Cocaine Bugs *See* Coke Bugs.

Cocaine Freebase Cocaine that has been highly purified and that produces an exhilarating effect when smoked. Freebase is an intermediate compound in the preparation of cocaine hydrochloride from coca. Freebase is derived by heating cocaine in a solvent such as ether. Without freebasing, cocaine has minimal psychoactive effects when smoked. The freebase is less susceptible than regular cocaine to decomposition when heated.

Cocaine Hydrochloride 1. Street cocaine. 2. The substance from which cocaine freebase is prepared.

Cocaine Kit Cocaine paraphernalia involving vials for storage, spoons for placing to-be-inhaled cocaine into, mirrors for pouring cocaine onto, and razor blades to scrape powdered cocaine into a "line" so that it can be sniffed with a straw.

Cocaine Test Kit Paraphernalia for testing presence of cocaine.

Cocainist Chronic cocaine user.

Cocainized Under the influence of cocaine.

Cocanuts Cocaine.

Cocarion Mixture of cocaine and heroin.

Cock Pipe Penis-shaped pipe used to smoke marihuana.

Cocktail Marihuana butt placed into the end of a tobacco cigarette.

Coconut Cocaine.

Cod Cock Mixture of codeine and some other medicine.

CODAP *See* Client Oriented Data Acquisition Process.

Codeine One of the main psychoactive substances in opium. Chemical name is methylmorphine. Isolated in 1832. Comes in the form of pills or liquid. Generally used as a pain reliever and cough suppressant, but also can produce euphoria. Classified as a narcotic. Tolerance and dependence can result from frequent usage. Sometimes used as a substitute for other opiates when they are unavailable.

Coffee LSD.

Coffee Habit Irregular use of narcotics. *Same as* Chipping.

Coke Cocaine.

Coke and Crystal Combination of cocaine and alcohol.

Coke Bugs Hallucinations resulting from chronic cocaine use, consisting of hallucinations that insects are crawling on or under the skin.

Coke Fiend Frequent and heavy user of cocaine.

Coke Freak Frequent and heavy user of cocaine.

Coke Head Frequent cocaine user.

Coke Oven 1. Place where cocaine users congregate to use cocaine together. 2. Place where cocaine is obtained.

Coke Party Gathering of cocaine users.

Coke Run Intensive use of drug over a relatively short period.

Coke Whore Cocaine user who does not buy his or her own drug but relies on others for free gifts.

Coked Under the influence of cocaine.

Coked Out Physically exhausted as a result of frequent use of cocaine.

Coked Up Under the influence of cocaine.

Cokey, Cokie Cocaine user.

Cokomo Cocaine user.

Cola 1. Flowering tops of marihuana plant. 2. Cocaine.

Cold and Hot Combination of cocaine and heroin.

Cold Shot Injection of counterfeit narcotics.

Cold Turkey Abrupt withdrawal from narcotics without being eased from them by other pharmacological agents such as methadone. One suggested origin for the expression is the appearance of gooseflesh associated with withdrawal in this way.

Coli Marihuana.

Collar 1. To arrest someone. 2. The stuffing between the medicine dropper and needle used to inject narcotics.

Collared Arrested.

Colombian Potent marihuana from Colombia. Comes in various colors, for example, gold, red. The colors have nothing to do with potency but are due to loss of green-colored chlorophyll. Absence of green color reveals the influence of various resins contained in marihuana, each of which has a color of its own. Colors may also be due to nutritional deficiencies experienced by the plant, for example, red indicates phosphorus deficiency; yellow, potassium deficiency. Color may also come from the material holding the marihuana together, for example, honey.

Colombian Gold Gold-colored marihuana from Colombia. *See* Colombian.

Colombian Red Red-colored marihuana from Colombia. *See* Colombian.

Colombo *Same as* Colombian.

Columbo PCP.

Columbus Black Marihuana from Ohio, black in color.

Come Down Final effects of a drug experience, often involving depression.

Come Home *Same as* Come Down.

Commercial Marihuana or hashish sold to buyers in contrast to higher-potency marihuana used by dealers for their own enjoyment.

Commission of Inquiry into the Nonmedical Use of Drugs Canadian commission convened to examine and evaluate illicit drug use in the 1970s. Also known as the LeDain Commission after its chairman, Gerald LeDain.

Comprehensive Drug Abuse Prevention and Control Act of 1970 U.S. code of laws regulating penalties for possession and use of illicit drugs. This law replaced the Harrison Narcotics Control Act of 1915. Title II of the Comprehensive Drug Act is called the Controlled Substances Act, and assigns various drugs to different schedules. Violation of the laws forbidding manufacturing, distribution, or disposal can result in a prison term of up to 15 years for a first offense and a fine of $5,000. For a second offense, penalties include prison term of up to 30 years and a fine of $50,000. Mandatory minimum sentences for users were abolished. The law was signed by President Nixon in 1970 and went into effect in 1971. The law replaced previous drug laws concerning narcotics and "dangerous drugs," such as the Boggs, Harrison, and Marihuana Tax acts.

Compulsive use Nonvoluntary use of drugs. Continued use is necessary to prevent withdrawal or other discomfort.

Con To cheat or deceive.

Conga Potent marihuana from Africa.

Congo Brown Potent marihuana from Africa, brown in color.

Congo Mataby Potent marihuana from Africa.

Connect To locate or buy drugs.

Connection 1. Drug seller. 2. Third major dealer in heroin trafficking, after importer and kilo connection. 3. Procurement of drugs.

Connector Drug seller.

Constitutional *Same as* Eyeopener.

Contact Drug seller.

Contact High Intoxicated from breathing marihuana smoke exhaled by others.

Contact Lens LSD solution on paper.

Controlled substance Drug listed in the Controlled Substance Act.

Controlled Substance Act Part of the Comprehensive Drug Abuse Prevention and Control Act of 1970. This Act provided five categories or "schedules" for psychoactive drugs, depending on the perceived harmfulness, abuse potential, and accepted medical usage. Heroin, LSD, and marihuana are included under Schedule 1, which means that they have the highest potential for abuse, highest dependence liability, and no currently accepted medical usage. Schedule 2 includes drugs such as morphine, methadone, and amphetamines—drugs that have approved medical usage. Drugs in Schedules 3, 4, and 5 have more widely recognized medical usage and less abuse potential.

Convert New narcotics user.

Cook 1. *Same as* Chef. 2. To prepare heroin for injection by dissolving it in water. This is done by placing the drug and some water in a spoon or bottle top and heating it over a small flame until the heroin goes into solution. 3. To prepare opium for smoking. 4. Pharmacist who sells drugs without a prescription. 5. Underground chemist who manufactures drugs illegally.

Cook a Pill To prepare opium for smoking.

Cook It Up To prepare heroin for injection.

Cooked 1. Under the influence of marihuana. 2. Dependent on narcotics.

Cooker 1. Spoon or bottle top used to dissolve heroin in water when it is heated. 2. Opium user who prepares his own opium for smoking.

Cookie 1. Opium user. 2. Cocaine. 3. Cocaine user.

Cooking Spoon Spoon used to dissolve heroin in water in preparation for intravenous administration.

Cool 1. In control. 2. Indifferent; aloof. 3. Smart; aware; knowledgeable.

Cool It To stop.

Cooler Jail.

Coolie Mud Low-potency opium.

Coozie Stash Drugs hidden in the vagina.

Cop 1. Police officer. 2. To buy; steal; take. 3. To admit to something.

Cop a Buy To buy drugs.

Cop a Fix To buy narcotics.

Cop a Match To buy a small amount of marihuana.

Cop a Plea To plead guilty to a lesser crime in order to receive a lighter sentence rather than contesting a more serious charge, and, if found guilty, receiving a harsher sentence.

Cop Man Drug seller.

Cop Out 1. To give up; back out at the last minute. 2. To plead guilty. 3. To stop using drugs.

Co-pilot *Same as* Babysitter.

Co-pilot Ben Benzedrine.

Co-pilots Amphetamines.

Coral Mickey Finn—mixture of alcohol and chloral hydrate.

Corgy Heroin.

Corine, Corrine Cocaine.

Cotickery Place where narcotics are bought.

Cotics Narcotics.

Coties Narcotics.

Cotton Small piece of cotton placed in the spoon or cooker in which heroin is dissolved and which is used as a filter in drawing the solution into the syringe.

Cotton Brothers Paraphernalia for intravenous injection. *Same as* Artillery.

Cotton Fever Fever accompanied by chills following use of unsanitary cotton to filter heroin.

Cotton Habit Sharing narcotics supply with others due to inability to pay for full dose.

Cotton Head *Same as* Cotton Shooter.

Cotton Picker *Same as* Cotton Shooter.

Cotton Shooter Destitute narcotics user who soaks the cotton used to filter narcotics in order to obtain any residual drug.

Cotton Top *Same as* Cotton Shooter.

Counterculture Cultural movement of the late 1960s and early 1970s in which participants rejected prevailing standards and authority and lived by their own standards. A significant component of this movement was exploration of consciousness through the use of drugs.

Courage Pills 1. Heroin in tablet form. 2. Barbiturates.

Courting Cecile Dependent on morphine.

Cowboy Independent drug seller.

Coyote Dishonest drug seller.

Cozmos PCP.

Crack a Script To get drugs from a pharmacist with a stolen prescription.

Crackers 1. LSD. 2. Amyl nitrite capsules.

Crank Methamphetamine.

Crank Bugs Imaginary bugs crawling over skin as a result of methamphetamine use.

Crank Commando Chronic methamphetamine user.

Cranking Repetitive use of methamphetamine.

Cranks Amphetamines.

Crap Low-potency heroin.

Crash 1. Unpleasant feeling resulting from drug usage. 2. To enter someone's home to stay for a short time. 3. To fall asleep after drug use.

Crash Pad Place to stay during last phases of drug experience.

Crater Large abscess in the skin caused by frequent injection into the area.

Crazy 1. Under the influence of marihuana. Term current during the 1940s. 2. Exceptional; excellent; good.

Creep Narcotics user who begs or does menial jobs to satisfy his drug needs.

Creep Joint *See* Creeper Joint.

Creeper Marihuana.

Creeper Joint Place where marihuana smoker is robbed while under the influence of the drug. Term current during the 1940s. Also referred to place where men were lured by prostitutes and then robbed.

Crink Methamphetamine.

Cripple Marihuana cigarette.

Cristal PCP.

Cristina Methamphetamine.

Cris Methamphetamine.

Croaker 1. Physician. 2. Physician who gives prescriptions for illicit drugs to drug users. 3. Prison physician.

Croaker Joint Hospital.

Crock 1. Opium pipe. 2. An alcoholic.

Cross Tops Amphetamines.

Crosses Amphetamines. *See* Catholic Aspirin.

Crossroads Amphetamines. *See* Catholic Aspirin.

Cross-tolerance Condition in which use of one drug conveys tolerance to one or more other drugs. For example, tolerance to heroin results in tolerance to methadone; tolerance to alcohol results in tolerance to Valium and barbiturates.

Crowd Overweight narcotics user.

Crown Crap Heroin.

Cruse Opium container.

Crusher Police officer.

Crystal 1. PCP. 2. Methamphetamine.

Crutch Device used to hold a burning marihuana cigarette butt.

Crystal Joint Marihuana to which PCP has been added.

Crystal Palace Place where methedrine is used.

Crystal Points PCP.

Crystal Ship Syringe containing methamphetamine.

Crystal T PCP.

Crystal Weed Marihuana to which PCP has been added.

Crystalized Under the influence of methamphetamine.

Crystals 1. Methamphetamine. 2. PCP.

Cube 1. LSD. 2. Gram of hashish. 3. Morphine.

Cube Head Frequent user of LSD.

Cube Juice Morphine.

Cubes LSD-impregnated sugar cubes.

Cucaracha, La Battle hymn of the Mexican revolution under Pancho Villa. The song later became popular in the United States. The song is about the cockroach's inability to walk without marihuana, but few Americans realized it at the time.

Culiacan Potent marihuana from Mexico.

Cum Brand name for amyl nitrite.

Cupcakes LSD.

Cured Marihuana soaked in sugar water and then dried. Purpose is to increase its weight.

Cushion Vein into which narcotics are injected.

Cut 1. To adulterate a drug. 2. Inert material added to a drug in order to increase its bulk.

Cutered Pill Opium pill from bottom of opium-pipe bowl that has become too hot.

CWP Marihuana cigarette holder.

Cyclazocine Narcotic antagonist.

Cyclones PCP.

D

D 1. Doriden. 2. Dilaudid. 3. LSD. 4. Dope.

D.A. Narcotics user.

Dabble To use narcotics intermittently.

Dabbling Intermittent use of narcotics.

Dagga Marihuana. Term originated in South Africa.

Dangerous drugs Legal term used prior to 1965 in reference to nonnarcotic drugs which were still under control, such as amphetamines, barbiturates. Term has now been replaced by *controlled substances*.

DARP Drug Abuse Reporting Program. Program begun in 1968 to keep track of admissions and progress of individuals being treated at federally funded institutes. Information is entered into computer research file located at Texas Christian University. The program provides basic information about patients and the outcome of treatment.

Darvon Propoxyphene napsylate. Pain reliever related to methadone. Originally thought to be nonaddicting. Comes in the form of pink oval pills, or capsules with red bodies and gray or pink caps. Not included in controlled substances schedules.

Datura *Datura stramonium*. Common names are jimsonweed, stinkweed, devil's apple, and thorn apple. Related to the potato family (Solanaceae), which also includes belladonna.

Dawamesc Favorite hashish confection of Club des Haschischins. Contains various ingredients, including hashish, pistachios, cinnamon, sugar, orange juice, cloves, and nutmeg.

DAWN *See* Drug Abuse Warning Network.

Day Care Alcohol or drug treatment program in which patients remain at a clinic during the day and return home at night.

Daytop Village Drug Addiction Treatment for Probationers. Therapeutic community for drug use rehabilitation located on Staten Island, New York. Serves as a halfway house to integrate former drug users into the community. Established in 1963.

DEA *See* Drug Enforcement Agency.

Dead Bang Injection of an inert material thought to be narcotics.

Deadly nightshade Belladonna.

Deadwood Undercover police officer posing as a drug user.

Deal Transaction involving drugs.

Deal in Weight To sell heroin in large quantities.

Dealer Drug seller. A dealer is often distinguished from a pusher in that a dealer sells "soft" drugs like marihuana, whereas a pusher sells "hard" drugs like heroin.

Dealer in Weight Heroin seller who buys from connection and sells to street dealer. The first distributor who may also be a heroin user.

Dealer's Band Rubber band worn around the wrist. Band holds heroin packets and is tied in such a way that the packets can be easily discarded if arrest is imminent.

Dealing Selling drugs.

Death Needle Thin steel rod on which opium is cooked before it is placed in bowl to smoke. *Same as* Yen Hock.

Death Trip Combination of LSD and datura.

Debris Marihuana particles, for example, seeds and stems, left after cleaning.

Deck 1. Pack of marihuana cigarettes. 2. Small packet of heroin.

Decriminalization Revision of drug laws such that certain offenses would be considered misdemeanors instead of felonies, thereby reducing punishment. Reduction of penalties for possession of small amounts of drugs such as marihuana is a component of the decriminalization movement. As originally proposed by the National Commission on Marihuana and Drug Abuse in 1972, private possession of marihuana would be legal whereas possession in public would be a misdemeanor.

Deeda LSD.

Deep Breath Spasms Regular time of day at which opium smoker has his drug.

Deliriant Any substance producing delusions or hallucinations.

Delirium Temporary state of mental disturbance with confusion, incoherence, or hallucinations.

Delirium tremens Last stage of withdrawal from alcohol.

Delta–9-tetrahydrocannabinol D⁹THC, the principal active ingredient in marihuana. The amount of THC contained in the marihuana plant depends on plant strain, climate, soil conditions, and method of harvesting. Different parts of the marihuana plant contain different amounts of THC. Generally, the parts of the plant highest above the ground contain the greatest amount of THC.

Delusion Belief not founded on evidence.

Delysid LSD. Trade name for the drug marketed by Sandoz drug company.

Demerol Meperidine hydrochloride, synthetic narcotic. Often used as an analgesic in childbirth.

Demerol test Field test for suspected Demerol. Suspected drug is placed in test tube and cobalt thiocyanate is added. If solution turns intense blue, substance contains Demerol.

Demis Demerol.

Den John Individual who earns money in an opium den by manually removing fecal material from rectums of constipated opium users.

Dependence Condition occurring as a result of continual use of certain drugs. Dependence can be either physical, psychological, or both. Physical dependence (addiction) is an adaptation of the body to the presence of a drug, such that its absence precipitates a withdrawal syndrome. Psychological dependence is a condition in which the user feels a desire, but not a compulsion, to continue drug use for a sense of well-being and feels discomfort when deprived of it. There is little tendency to increase the dosage in connection with psychological dependence.

Depersonalization Loss of sense of self.

Depressant Drug that reduces activity of bodily organs, especially the brain; for example, alcohol, barbiturates, tranquilizers. Effects are dose-related and progress from decreased anxiety, to sedation, sleep, anesthesia, coma, and death.

Desbutal Trade name for a compound containing both an amphetamine (methamphetamine hydrochloride) and a barbiturate (pentobarbital sodium).

Deserpidine Naturally occurring compound found in *Rauwolfia ser-*

pentina, the snake-root plant, which is used in several antipsycotic drugs, such as Harmonyl.

Desipramine hydrochloride Antidepressant drug. Trade name is Pertofrane or Norpramin.

Desoxyn Trade name for methamphetamine hydrochloride.

Dessicator Pipe used to smoke freebase cocaine.

Destroyed Physically or psychologically exhausted and unable to cope as a result of drug use.

Detox Center, Detoxification Center Place where treatment is provided while individual undergoes detoxification.

Detoxication, Detoxification Treatment program whereby an individual who is dependent on a drug is withdrawn from it under medical supervision. The symptoms associated with the withdrawal depend on the type of drug used and the amount of time the individual has been using the drug. In the case of heroin dependence, the patient is gradually weaned from the drug by administering methadone and then gradually reducing the dosage of that drug. In the case of alcohol dependence, Librium is often given in conjunction with withdrawal.

Detroit Pink PCP.

Deuce Two drug capsules, usually amphetamines or barbiturates.

Deuce Bag Two dollars' worth of a drug, usually marihuana.

Deuce Someone To sell someone two marihuana cigarettes.

Devil's Dust PCP.

Dew Marihuana.

Dex Dexedrine.

Dexamyl Trade name for drug containing an amphetamine (dextroamphetamine sulfate) and a barbiturate (amobarbital).

Dexedrine Trade name for dextroamphetamine sulfate.

Dexies Dexedrine.

Dexo Dexedrine.

Dextroamphetamine sulfate Amphetamine compound manufactured as Dexedrine.

Dextromoramide Synthetic narcotic analgesic.

Dexy Dexedrine.

Diacetylmorphine Chemical name for heroin.

Diazepam Chemical name for Valium, an antianxiety tranquilizer and muscle relaxant.

Dibenzopyran system Chemical notation for describing cannabinoids.

Did the Mail Come? Did you get the drugs?

Dig To understand.

Dihydrocodeine Semisynthetic narcotic derivative of morphine.

Dilaudid Trade name for hydromorphone hydrochloride, semisynthetic derivative of morphine. Has greater potency than morphine but is not as constipating, produces less nausea, has a shorter duration of action, and withdrawal is less severe. Sold in the form of capsules, tablets, or in cough syrup.

Dille-Koppanyi test Field test for barbiturates. Suspected material from capsule or tablet is placed in test tube and cobalt acetate is added followed by isopropylamine. If red-violet color results, barbiturates are present.

Dillies Dilaudid.

Dilocol Cough syrup containing hydromorphone hydrochloride. *See* Dilaudid.

Dilutant Inert material used to increase the bulk of an active substance without affecting its activity.

Dime Ten dollars.

Dime Bag Ten dollars' worth of drugs.

Dime of Buzz Amount of PCP that can be put on a coffee stirrer spoon. About 50 milligrams.

Dimethoxymethamphetamine (DOM) Hallucinogen related in its chemical structure to amphetamine and mescaline. Also known as STP.

Dimethyltryptamine (DMT) Hallucinogen with effects similar to LSD.

Ding, Dingbat Marihuana.

Dinghiyen Hypodermic syringe.

Dingus Homemade hypodermic syringe.

Dinky Dow Marihuana cigarette. Term used by American soldiers in Vietnam.

Dip Narcotics user.

Dip and Dab Irregular use of narcotics.

Diphenyldydramine hydrochloride Antianxiety tranquilizer. Trade name is Benadryl.

Diphenylhydantoin Anticonvulsant used to control epilepsy. One of the top twenty drugs used for psychoactive effects that result in emergency room treatment.

Dipped Dependent on narcotics.

Dipper PCP.

Diprenorphine Narcotic antagonist.

Dirt Grass Low-potency marihuana.

Dirty 1. Uncleaned marihuana; contains seeds, stems, and leaves. 2. Possessing marihuana or any other drug.

Dirty Urine Urine specimen in which drugs have been detected.

Distribution Channel Chain of heroin distribution from importation to street sale. Chain consists of importer, kilo connection, connection, dealer in weight, street dealer, juggler.

Ditch Joint in the arm above the elbow where narcotics users initially begin injecting drugs intravenously.

Ditch Weed Marihuana.

Ditran Piperidyl benzilate, a hallucinogen.

Diversion Nonpunitive method of dealing with drug offenders whereby they are given the opportunity to participate in a treatment program after arrest rather than face trial and possible imprisonment. Prosecution is deferred during participation in the program, and upon completion charges are often dismissed.

DMT Dimethyltryptamine, hallucinogen structurally similar to psilocin. Psilocin is the compound into which psilocybin, the psychoactive constituent of certain hallucinogen-producing mushrooms, is converted. Considered to be easily synthesized. DMT is often placed on oregano or parsley and smoked.

DOA PCP. Abbreviation for dead on arrival.

Do To take drugs.

Do a Brody *See* Brody.

Do a Figure Eight *See* Figure eight.

Do a Joint To smoke marihuana.

Do a Line Sniff powdered PCP or cocaine.

Do a Line of Buzz To sniff PCP.

Do It Now Foundation Nonprofit foundation concerned with prevention of drug abuse.

Do Right John Narcotics user.

Do Righter Non–drug user.

Do Up 1. To smoke marihuana. 2. To inject heroin intravenously.

Doctor To alter the potency of a drug.

Doctor White Cocaine.

Dodo Narcotics user.

Dog PCP.

Dog Food Heroin.

Dog Tag Prescription for narcotics.

Dogie, Doojee, Duji Heroin.

Doing Your Business Smoking marihuana.

Doll 1. Barbiturates. 2. Any kind of pill.

Dollies Dolophine.

Dolly Dolophine.

Dolophine Trade name for methadone.

DOM Dimethoxymethamphetamine, a potent hallucinogen related in its chemical structure to amphetamine and mescaline. Also called STP, from the motor oil additive, supposed to enhance engine performance.

Domes LSD. Term possibly derived from effects on the brain, which is also called the dome.

Dominos Amphetamines.

Dona Juanita Marihuana.

Donjem Marihuana.

Doobie Marihuana.

Doojee Heroin.

Dool Someone dependent on narcotics.

Dopamine Chemical that is involved in transmission of information between nerves and is an intermediate compound in the production of the neurochemical norepinephrine.

Dopatorium Place where narcotics are used.

Dope 1. Any drug. Most popular term for marihuana in 1970s. Prior to that it was most popular term for heroin. 2. To add alcohol or another drug to a drink.

Dope Cop Federal narcotics officer.

Dope Den Old expression referring to place where heroin and, later, marihuana were taken.

Dope Fiend Narcotics addict. Term used primarily in the 1930s and 1940s.

Dope Fighter Narcotics user.

Dope Gun Hypodermic syringe.

Dope Head Frequent marihuana smoker.

Dope Hop Someone dependent on narcotics.

Dope Jag Under the influence of narcotics.

Dope Lawyer Attorney who specializes in defending persons accused of violating drug laws.

Dope Peddler Narcotics seller.

Dope Pimp Narcotics seller who gives drugs to potential users free of charge to create dependence so that they will later buy from him.

Dope Pipe Pipe for smoking marihuana or hashish.

Dope Ring Gang smuggling or selling narcotics.

Dope Runner Intermediary between narcotics seller and user.

Dope Smoke 1. Marihuana. 2. Hashish.

Doped Cigarettes Marihuana.

Doper 1. Marihuana smoker. 2. Frequent user of psychoactive drugs.

Doperie Opium den.

Dopester *Same as* Doper.

Dopey Under the influence of a drug.

Dopium Opium.

Doriden Nonbarbiturate sedative/hypnotic drug.

Dose, Dosage The amount of drug taken or administered.

Dose-effect, Dose-response relationship Relationship between the amount of drug taken and the effect it produces.

Dot Dose of LSD.

Double Dipper PCP.

Double Header Two marihuana cigarettes smoked at the same time. Purpose is to increase the amount of smoke inhaled.

Double Trouble Tuinal, a sedative containing two barbiturates— amobarbital and secobarbital.

Double-blind study Procedure involving drug research in which neither the experimenter nor the subject knows beforehand whether an inert substance or an active drug is being given to the subject. This procedure is implemented to minimize biased assessments of drug effects.

Douche Intravenous injection of narcotics.

Down 1. Unpleasant aftereffects of drug use. 2. Returning to normal state following marihuana use.

Down to the Cotton So desperate for narcotics that the user soaks the cotton used to filter narcotics to obtain any residual drug.

Downer 1. Depressant drug. 2. Unpleasant experience.

Downer Freak Chronic barbiturate user.

Downies Barbiturates.

Downs *Same as* Downer.

Downtown Heroin.

DPT Diphenyl tryptamine, a hallucinogen.

Dr. Bananas Brand name for amyl nitrite.

Dr. Feelgood Physician who gives prescriptions for illicit drugs to drug users.

Dr. White Narcotics.

Drag 1. Deep inhalation of tobacco or marihuana cigarette. 2. Boring, unpleasant situation.

Drag Weed Marihuana.

Dragged State of anxiety sometimes experienced after smoking marihuana.

Dream 1. Opium. 2. Cocaine.

Dream Beads Opium.

Dream Boat Place where narcotics are sold to users.

Dream Gum Opium.

Dream Pipe Opium pipe.

Dream Stick 1. Marihuana cigarette. 2. Opium. 3. Opium pipe.

Dream Stuff Narcotics.

Dream Wax Opium.

Dreamer Morphine user.

Dreams Narcotics.

Drink Molten Lead To undergo withdrawal from narcotics.

Drink Texas Tea To smoke marihuana.

Dripper Homemade hypodermic syringe usually consisting of an eyedropper to which a pin is attached.

Drivers Amphetamines.

Drop 1. To swallow a drug. 2. To deliver drugs to a buyer.

Drop a Dime To inform on someone.

Drop a Joint To smoke a marihuana cigarette.

Drop a Rack To swallow, all at once, several different drugs in pill or capsule form.

Drop a Roll *Same as* Drop a Rack.

Drop Man Person who delivers drugs to buyers. Usually a nonuser.

Drop Out To detach oneself from everyday concerns.

Drop Shot Intravenous injection of a drug.

Dropper Medicine dropper used as a syringe to administer heroin intravenously.

Drug 1. Although usually thought of as any substance used to treat disease, a more proper definition is any substance that affects bodily function, including any material—plant, powder, fluid, solid, or gas—that can be eaten, drunk, injected, sniffed, inhaled, or absorbed from the skin. 2. Substance that affects the body and is taken for other than medically prescribed reasons.

Drug abuse Nontherapeutic use of drugs to the point where it affects the health of the individual or impacts adversely on others. The term is very subjective.

Drug Abuse Act of 1970 *See* Comprehensive Drug Abuse Prevention and Control Act of 1970.

Drug Abuse Control Amendment of 1965 An amendment to the food and drug laws whereby drugs such as amphetamines, barbiturates and hallucinogens were designated as "dangerous drugs" and were placed under federal control. Also called the Harris-Dodd Act. The purpose of the law was to gain better control of illegal manufacture and sale of these drugs.

Drug Abuse Council Nonprofit foundation located in Washington, D.C., aimed at providing information about drug abuse. No longer in existence.

Drug Abuse Warning Network (DAWN) Program sponsored by the Bureau of Narcotics and Dangerous Drugs to provide information about the adverse effects of drugs. Basic information is derived from institutes that have contact with emergency-related reactions to drug use, e.g., crisis centers, hospital emergency rooms. Program is now administered by the Drug Enforcement Administration.

Drug addict The most popular term for a narcotics user. Now extended to mean any chronic user of psychoactive drugs.

Drug Booster *Same as* Dope Pimp.

Drug Culture Group of people whose patterns of behavior involve and are supportive of recreational use of drugs.

Drug Enforcement Agency (DEA) Created in 1973 by President Nixon by merging BNDD and ODALE. Currently the main federal agency concerned with enforcement of drug laws.

Drug misuse Using a drug more frequently than warranted, or taking amounts that are greater than initially prescribed.

Drug Partisan Narcotics user.

Drug Policy Office One of the three main agencies responsible for determining federal drug policy. The other such agencies are the Drug Enforcement Administration and the National Institute on Drug Abuse. The Drug Policy Office is solely concerned with drug abuse policy and is part of the White House Domestic Policy Staff, which assists the president in determining, coordinating, and monitoring domestic and international activities for all executive agencies.

Drug Scene Subculture of drug use.

Druggie, Druggy College student who frequently uses psychoactive drugs and has experimented widely with many different such drugs.

Drunk 1. Intoxicated. Usually used in conjunction with alcohol, but, in the 1930s, also used in connection with other drugs, such as marihuana. 2. Someone intoxicated by alcohol.

Dry Not having had drugs.

Dry Booze Narcotics.

Dry Grog Narcotics.

Dry Whiskey Peyote.

Dubbe, Dubee, Dubie, Duby *Same as* Doobie.

Duct Cocaine.

Duffy *Same as* Brody.

Dug Out Narcotics user who has alienated all friends and who has no resources.

Dugee, Dugie, Duji Heroin.

Duke In To expose an undercover police officer.

Dumb Smuggler Animal used to smuggle drugs. Drugs are fed to animal and it is later killed and drug is removed.

Dummy Inert material sold as heroin.

Dummy Dust PCP.

Duquenois test Forensic test used to detect presence of marihuana. Test substance is mixed with vanillin, acetaldehyde, alcohol, and hydrochloric acid. If marihuana is present, the mixture turns violet.

Dust 1. Powdered narcotics. 2. Cocaine. 3. PCP. 4. To add a drug, e.g., PCP, to another, e.g., marihuana. *See* Dust Joint.

Dust Joint Marihuana cigarette to which PCP has been added.

Dust of Angels PCP.

Dust of Morpheus Powdered morphine.

Dusted Dependent on narcotics.

Duster 1. Tobacco or marihuana cigarette to which heroin has been added. 2. Tobacco or marihuana cigarette to which PCP has been added.

Dusting Adding heroin or other drugs to a marihuana cigarette.

Dutch courage Courage brought on by drinking alcohol or use of drugs.

Dutch Mill 1. Place where narcotics are sold to users. 2. Place where narcotics are used.

Dynamite 1. Potent marihuana or other drug. 2. Extraordinarily good; superlative. Originally used in reference to narcotics. 3. Narcotics. 4. Combination of heroin and cocaine.

Dynamite Stocks Methamphetamine.

Dynamiter Narcotics user.

Dynamiters Potent marihuana cigarettes.

Dyno Relatively undiluted heroin.

Dysphoria Opposite of euphoria; sense of uneasiness, unpleasantness, sadness.

E

Ear Rings Sensation of ringing in the ear associated with use of cocaine freebase.

Easing Powder Narcotics.

Eater Narcotics user who takes his drug orally.

Eating Poppy Seed Cakes Dependent on opium.

Echoes Flashback—reoccurrence of a drug experience long after drug use.

Efficacy Ability of a drug to produce a desired effect.

Eighth One-eighth of an ounce or gram.

Elbow Pound of marihuana.

Electric Butter Marihuana sauteed in butter.

Electric Kool Aid Punch drink to which LSD has been added.

Elephant, Elephant Tranquilizers PCP.

Elevation Opium.

Em, Emm Morphine.

Embalming Fluid PCP.

Embroidery Scars on the skin resulting from injection.

Emergency Gun Makeshift hypodermic consisting of a medicine dropper and a pin. The skin is punctured and the solution is injected from the dropper.

Emetic Substance that causes vomiting.

Emsel Morphine.

Endorphins Opioid substances produced by the body that resemble opiates in many of the effects they produce.

Energizer PCP.

Engine 1. Narcotics paraphernalia. 2. Opium pipe.

Enkephalins Group of endorphin chemicals.

Equanil Meprobamate, an antianxiety tranquilizer.

Ergogenics Stimulants.

Erth PCP.

Estuffa Heroin.

Ethanol Alcohol.

Ethchlorvynol Nonbarbiturate sedative/hypnotic. Trade name is Placidyl.

Ether Base Cocaine freebase using ether as a solvent.

Ethinamate Nonbarbiturate sedative/hypnotic. Trade name is Valmid.

Euphoria Sense of well-being, happiness, pleasure. Main reason for use of many drugs is to achieve this state.

Euphoriant Drug causing euphoria.

Every Mother's Blood Combination of hallucinogens.

Experience LSD experience.

Experimenter Occasional user of LSD.

Explorer's Club Group of LSD users.

Eye Dropper Medicine dropper attached to a hypodermic needle as a substitute syringe.

Eye Opener 1. First drink of alcohol or use of drug of the day. 2. Amphetamines.

E-Z Wider First specially designed rolling paper for making marihuana cigarettes. These papers are wider than traditional cigarette papers.

F

Faced *See* Shit-faced.

Factory 1. Paraphernalia for injection of narcotics. 2. Distribution point where drug pushers obtain their supplies. 3. Clandestine laboratory where illicit drugs are manufactured.

Fagan Informer.

Faggot Marihuana.

Fairy Powder Narcotics in powder form.

Fake Medicine dropper. The substitute syringe used with a needle to give an injection.

Fake a Blast 1. To pretend to inhale marihuana cigarette. 2. To pretend to become intoxicated.

Fake Aloo Homemade hypodermic syringe.

Fake STP PCP.

Fakes Counterfeit drugs.

Fall 1. To be arrested. 2. To be sentenced to jail.

Fall Out To fall asleep after smoking marihuana. 2. Sensations from drug use.

False negative Results from a test which indicate the absence of something when in fact it is present. For example, in a drug screening test, a false negative result would suggest the absence of a drug when it is actually present. Such errors arise due to insensitive test procedures, poorly performed procedures, problems in collection, storage, or transport of samples, or clerical errors.

False positive The opposite of false negative, that is, a drug test in which the results suggest the presence of a drug when in fact it is not present.

Famine Absence of drugs due to crackdown by police.

Fancy Chef Good opium cook.

Fang Narcotics injection.

Fang It To inject narcotics.

Far Out 1. Excellent; superior. 2. Unusual; remarkable; sensational.

Farmer 1. Non-drug user. 2. Naive person; a "square."

Fat 1. Thick. 2. Possessing a large amount of marihuana.

Fat Jay Thick marihuana cigarette, thickened because of low potency.

Fat Joint *Same as* Fat Jay.

Fatty Thick marihuana cigarette.

Fay Hound Homosexual marihuana user.

Feathered Under the influence of narcotics.

Fed Federal narcotics agent.

Federal Beef Federal narcotics offense.

Federal Bureau of Narcotics First (1930) federal agency specifically organized to control illicit drugs. The Federal Bureau of Narcotics was initially responsible for enforcement of the Harrison Narcotic Act (1915). Powers were based on federal taxing powers and therefore the agency was part of the treasury department. The bureau was abolished in 1968 and replaced by the Bureau of Narcotics and Dangerous Drugs (BNDD). The BNDD was removed from the Treasury and made part of the Justice Department.

Federal Drug Abuse Policy Policy of the federal government regarding drug abuse. Currently policy is recommended by three agencies, the Drug Enforcement Administration (DEA), the Drug Policy Office, and the National Institute of Drug Abuse (NIDA).

Feeblo Narcotics user.

Feed Narcotics.

Feed and Grain Man Narcotics seller.

Feed Bag Container of narcotics.

Feed Store Place where drugs are sold.

Feed Your Head To take drugs orally.

Feeder Hypodermic syringe.

Feeding Taking narcotics.

Feeding Candy Taking cocaine.

Feel Like the World's Against Me Suffering from a lack of marihuana. 1930s expression.

Feel the Habit Early sensations of withdrawal from narcotics.

Feel the Thing Coming On *Same as* Feel the Habit.

Felony Any offense for which a sentence is to be served in a state or federal prison. Each state has its own definition.

Fence Middleman in sale of stolen merchandise.

Fennel Marihuana.

Fermentation Chemical changes by which alcohol is produced from naturally occurring substances such as fruit juice. Fermentation occurs usually as a result of yeasts acting, in conjunction with enzymes, on sugars.

Ferry Dust Heroin.

F-forties Seconal capsules. From the letter and number stamped on the capsule.

Field dependence Behavior determined by one's surroundings.

Fiend Drug addict; someone who cannot control his drug use.

Fifty LSD.

Fifty-cent Bag Fifty dollars' worth of marihuana.

Figure Eight To feign spasm associated with withdrawal in hopes of convincing a physician to administer or prescribe narcotics.

Fin 1. Five dollars. 2. Five-year jail sentence.

Fine Stuff Finely manicured marihuana.

Finger 1. Quantity of hashish about the size and shape of a finger. 2. Condom filled with narcotics which is then swallowed or placed in the rectum. 3. To inform on someone.

Finger Wave Rectal examination for hidden narcotics.

Fink 1. Informer; betrayer. 2. To inform.

Fir Hashish.

Fire To inject narcotics intravenously.

Fire Plug A large bolus of opium.

Fire Up 1. To light a marihuana cigarette; to smoke marihuana or hashish. 2. To inject narcotics.

First Baseman The first person to smoke cocaine freebase at a party. Often the person who prepared it, i.e., the Chef.

First Line Morphine.

Fit *See* Outfit.

Five-Cent Bag Five dollars' worth of drugs.

Fives Five-milligram tablets of amphetamines.

Fix 1. Injection of narcotics. 2. Narcotics.

Fix Me Sell me narcotics.

Fixed Under the influence of narcotics.

Flag 1. To arrest. 2. Appearance of blood in the hypodermic after the needle has been injected into a vein and the plunger has been drawn back. Indicates that needle is indeed in vein.

Flake 1. Cocaine. 2. Almost pure cocaine. 3. PCP. 4. To fall asleep from drug use.

Flake Acid LSD solution on paper.

Flash 1. Sudden feeling of euphoria from intravenous injection of heroin. 2. Sudden sensation felt in the stomach following injection of narcotics. 3. LSD.

Flashback To experience drug-associated feelings long after drug use. Usually mentioned in connection with LSD.

Flashing Sniffing glue or other solvents.

Flat Blues LSD.

Flats LSD.

Flattened Stuporous from drug use.

Flea Powder Low-potency narcotics.

Fledgling Novice narcotics user.

Flier Narcotics user.

Flip, Flip Out 1. To have an unpleasant experience following marihuana use, or conversely, to have an enjoyable reaction. 2. To inform. 3. To be rendered unconscious by a drink or drug that has been surreptitiously altered, such as a Mickey Finn. 4. Emotional disturbance from drug use, especially LSD or amphetamines.

Floating Light-headedness from smoking marihuana, drinking alcohol, or using narcotics.

Flogged Under the influence of a drug.

Flop To smoke opium.

Florida Snow Substitute cocaine, usually lidocaine.

Flowers Marihuana flowers.

Fluff 1. To chop heroin or cocaine to give it a finer consistency and more bulk. 2. To add mannite to heroin to inflate its volume.

Flunk Out To start using potent drugs.

Flush Sensation of intense euphoria resulting from drug use.

Flushing Drawing blood back into the syringe to make sure that a vein has been entered.

Fly agaric The mushroom *Amanita muscaria*. Main psychoactive ingredient is bufotenine.

Flyer Drug user.

Flying 1. Light-headed from smoking marihuana. 2. Intoxicated by a drug.

Flying Dutchman Narcotics seller.

Flying in the Clouds Under the influence of narcotics.

Flying Saucers Morning-glory seeds.

Foil Small packet of narcotics.

Fold Up To stop using narcotics.

Foo Foo Dust 1. Morphine. 2. Heroin. 3. Cocaine.

Foolish Powder 1. Cocaine. 2. Heroin. 3. Any drug.

Foon Opium pill prepared for smoking.

Football 1. Mescaline. 2. Amphetamines in oval capsules.

Foreign Mud Cooked opium.

Forensic medicine Application of medical disciplines to law.

Fortnightey Irregular narcotics user.

Forty-niner Habitual cocaine user.

Forwards Amphetamines.

Four and Doors *Same as* Four-doors.

Four-doors Combination of codeine and Doriden. Produces euphoria similar to low dose of heroin.

Fours Tylenol tablets containing codeine. Term derived from the number scored on the tablet.

Foxy Intuitive feeling from smoking marihuana.

Fractured Drunk; intoxicated.

Fraho, Frajo Marihuana cigarette.

Frame a Twister To feign withdrawal in hopes of convincing a physician to administer or prescribe narcotics.

Frantic Junk Stage Initial stages of withdrawal from narcotics.

Frazzled Drunk; intoxicated.

Freak 1. Habitual heavy user of drugs; user obsessed with drug use. 2. One who derives enjoyment out of both using drugs and being known as a habitual drug user. 3. Chronic drug user who exhibits bizarre behavior.

Freak House Place where methamphetamine users congregate to take drugs together.

Freak Out 1. To hallucinate. 2. To become stuporous. 3. To have an unpleasant reaction to a drug.

Freaky Bizarre.

Free Clinic Medical clinic providing medical treatment without charge, including treatment for drug-related problems.

Free Grass Marihuana remaining after most has been sold. Kept for seller's own use.

Free Smoke *Same as* Free Grass.

Free Trip To experience drug-associated feelings long after drug use. Usually mentioned in connection with LSD. *Same as* Flashback.

Freebase Purified cocaine. Intermediate compound in preparation of cocaine hydrochloride from coca. *See* Cocaine Freebase.

Freebase Conversion Kit Paraphernalia for preparing freebase. *See* Cocaine Freebase.

Freeze 1. To refuse to sell drugs. 2. Numbing sensation associated with snorting cocaine.

French Blue Combination of amphetamine and barbiturate.

French Quaalude Methaqualone.

Freon Freak Inhaler of propellant Freon.

Fresh and Sweet Just released from jail.

Freshen To start using narcotics.

Freshisy *Same as* Fresh and Sweet.

Fried Very intoxicated by a drug or alcohol.

Fried to the Gills *Same as* Fried.

Frisco Speedball Mixture of equal portions of heroin and cocaine. Sometimes LSD is also added.

Frisk Search.

Frisky Powder Cocaine.

From Mount Shasta Dependent on narcotics.

Front 1. To sell drugs on credit to another dealer. 2. To give payment before drug has been received.

Frost Freak *Same as* Freon freak.

Frosted Under the influence of cocaine.

Frosty *Same as* Frosted.

Frozen Very intoxicated by a drug.

Fruit Salad Variety of drugs contributed by a group and shared by them. Participants take them without knowing which drugs they are ingesting.

F-sixties Histadyl, an antihistamine.

F-sixty-sixes Tuinal with Seconal.

Fu Marihuana.

Fu Manchu Marihuana smoker.

Fuck the Hops To have dreams involving sex while under the influence of narcotics.

Fucked Up Unable to think or speak clearly, or to coordinate one's movements, as a result of drug use.

Fuel PCP.

Full Blast Very intoxicated by a drug.

Full Moon 1. Round cake of hashish. 2. Upper part of peyote cactus.

Full of Junk Under the influence of narcotics.

Full Time Life term in jail.

Fun Opium.

Fun Joint Opium den.

Fun Medicine Narcotics.

Funny Cigarettes Marihuana. Term used during 1930s and 1940s.

Funny Farm Psychiatric hospital.

Funny Stuff Marihuana.

Fur-lined Throat Dry throat of opium smoker, which can be relieved only by fruit juices.

Fuzz Police.

Fuzzy Drunk; intoxicated.

G

G Paper funnel placed into an eyedropper when pouring heroin into it for subsequent injection.

Gage, Gauge, Guage Marihuana. From *ganja*, the term used for marihuana in India and Jamaica.

Gage, Gauge, Guage Butt Marihuana cigarette.

Gage, Gauge, Guage Party Party at which marihuana is smoked.

Gage in the Rough Uncleaned marihuana.

Gaged Intoxicated by marihuana.

Gainesville Green Marihuana grown in Florida.

Gal Head Narcotics user.

Gallery Place where narcotics users congregate to inject themselves or be injected. *Same as* Shooting Gallery.

Galloping Horse Heroin.

Gammon Microgram.

Gammot 1. Morphine. 2. Heroin.

Gang, Gange Marihuana.

Ganger Narcotics.

Gangster Marihuana.

Gangster Pills Barbiturates.

Ganja Marihuana. Term originated in India and Jamaica.

Gap 1. Yawning and salivation associated with initial stages of narcotics withdrawal. 2. Money.

Gapper Narcotics user beginning to feel the onset of withdrawal.

Garbage Low-potency drugs.

Garbage Freak Polydrug user.

Garbage Head *Same as* Garbage Freak.

Gas 1. Good time; pleasing, amusing incident. 2. Nitrous oxide.

Gas Crystals Intermediate product formed in conversion of coca into cocaine hydrochloride.

Gasblaster Use of nitrous oxide after smoking cocaine freebase.

Gash Marihuana.

Gasket Piece of paper or cloth wedged between the end of a dropper and a needle to prevent air from being injected into a vein during intravenous narcotics injection.

Gasp To experience early feelings of withdrawal from narcotics.

Gasper Marihuana cigarette.

Gassed Intoxicated; euphoric.

Gassing Sniffing gasoline fumes.

Gate Vein into which narcotics are injected.

Gates Marihuana.

Gauge Marihuana.

Gauge Butt Marihuana cigarette.

Gauged Intoxicated by marihuana.

Gazer Federal narcotics officer.

G.B. Goof balls—barbiturates.

G.B.'s Barbiturates.

Gear Marihuana.

Geared Up Drunk; intoxicated.

Gee Opium.

Gee Bag 1. Strainer at base of opium-pipe bowl. 2. Packing used to make connection between opium-pipe bowl and stem airtight.

Gee Fat *Same as* Yen Shee.

Gee Gee Opium pipe.

Gee Head Paregoric user.

Gee Rag Cloth used to make connection between opium-pipe bowl and stem airtight.

Gee Stick Opium pipe.

Gee Yen Opium precipitate in the stem of an opium pipe.

Geed, Geeded, Gheed Up 1. Intoxicated by narcotics or alcohol. 2. Destitute narcotics user.

Geep *Same as* Gee Rag.

Geesed Drunk; intoxicated.

Geeser Small amount of narcotics.

Geez 1. Narcotics. 2. Narcotics injection.

Geezed *Same as* Geesed.

Geezer 1. Small amount of narcotics. 2. Narcotics injection.

Gelatin LSD solution on paper.

Gem Narcotics.

Generic name Chemical name for a drug as opposed to its trade name.

George 1. One dollar. 2. One-year jail sentence.

George Smack Potent heroin.

Geronimo Barbiturates dissolved in alcohol.

Get a Finger Wave *See* Finger Wave.

Get Down To smoke marihuana.

Get Fixed *See* Fixed.

Get in the Groove To begin to use drugs.

Get Narkied To begin to use narcotics.

Get Off To become intoxicated by a drug.

Get On *Same as* Get Down.

Get Over To use just enough of a drug to avoid withdrawal distress.

Get Righteous 1. To begin to experience sensations associated with withdrawal from narcotics.

Get Straight To take narcotics.

Get the Monkey off My Back To stop using narcotics.

Get the Sting To become dependent on narcotics.

Get the Use Of To become a narcotics user.

Get the Vulture off My Veins To stop using narcotics.

Get the Yen Off To take narcotics.

Get Through To buy drugs.

Get Up First use of drugs of the day. *See* Eye Opener.

Get Up Steam To drink alcohol and then inject narcotics or smoke marihuana.

Get with It To inject narcotics intravenously.

Get Your Nose Cold To sniff cocaine.

Ghost 1. LSD. 2. Opium smoker.

Ghow Opium.

Giggle Smoke Marihuana.

Giggle Weed Marihuana.

Gimmick Paraphernalia for intravenous injection. *Same as* Artillery.

Gin 1. Type of alcoholic beverage. 2. Cocaine.

Girl Cocaine.

Give Birth To evacuate the bowels following the constipating effects of narcotics.

Give Birth to a Duster To evacuate hard stools from the bowel.

Give Him His Wings To introduce someone to drug use.

Give Wings 1. To inject someone with narcotics. 2. To teach someone how to administer a self-injection of narcotics.

Glad Rag Cloth saturated with solvent to be inhaled.

Glad Stuff 1. Cocaine. 2. Morphine. 3. Opium.

Glass 1. Hypodermic syringe. 2. Methedrine in capsules.

Glass Eyes Narcotics user.

Glass Gun Hypodermic syringe.

Glassy-eyed Under the influence of narcotics. From the glassy stare following drug use.

Glom 1. To use drugs. 2. To take more than one's share of drug at a drug party.

Glory Seeds Morning-glory seeds.

Glue Sniffing Inhalation of glue products containing aromatic hydrocarbons such as toluene.

Glued Arrested.

Gluey Glue sniffer.

Glutethimide Nonbarbiturate sedative/hypnotic used to treat insomnia. Trade name is Doriden. Comes in the form of white tablet or blue and white capsule. Often used in combination with codeine. *See* Four-Doors.

G-man Federal narcotics agent.

Go Unspecified amount of narcotics.

Go in the Sewer To inject narcotics intravenously.

Go in the Skin To inject narcotics subcutaneously instead of intravenously.

Go Loco To smoke marihuana.

Go on a Sleigh Ride To use cocaine.

Go Straight To stop using drugs.

Go Up To take amphetamines.

God's Medicine Morphine.

Goies Amphetamines.

Going Downhill Feeling the final effects of narcotics withdrawal.

Going to Get the Laundry Out Going to smoke opium.

Going Up Taking amphetamines.

Gold Potent gold-colored marihuana, for example, Acapulco Gold, Colombian Gold, Kona Gold.

Gold Dust Cocaine.

Gold Leaf 1. Potent marihuana. 2. Acapulco Gold. 3. Marihuana originating from another country.

Gold Leaf Special Potent marihuana cigarette.

Golden Girl Potent cocaine.

Golden Triangle Major opium-producing area of the world (about 70 percent of world's illegal supply), consisting of northeastern Burma, northern Thailand, and northern Laos.

G.O.M. *Abbreviation for* God's own medicine—morphine.

Goma 1. Morphine. 2. Opium.

Gomade Moto Hashish.

Gone Under the influence of narcotics.

Gong 1. Opium pipe. 2. Opium smoker.

Gong Beater Opium user.

Gong Kicker 1. Opium user. 2. Marihuana user.

Gonga 1. Marihuana. 2. Intoxicated by opium.

Gonga Dust Morphine.

Gonga Smudge Marihuana cigarette.

Gonger 1. Opium. 2. Opium pipe. 3. Opium user.

Gonger Den Place where opium is used.

Gongo with a Jump *See* Mickey Finn.

Gongola Opium pipe.

Goober Marihuana cigarette.

Good Stuff High-quality drugs or alcohol.

Good Time Man Drug seller.

Goods Narcotics.

Goof Marihuana user.

Goof Artist 1. Barbiturate user. 2. Inhalant sniffer.

Goof Balls 1. Barbiturates. 2. Any drug in capsule form.

Goof Butt Marihuana cigarette.

Goofed (Up) Intoxicated by marihuana, barbiturates, or opium.

Goofer Barbiturate user.

Goofers Barbiturates.

Goofing 1. Smoking marihuana. 2. Teasing someone who is intoxicated on marihuana. 3. Under the influence of barbiturates.

Goofy Dust Cocaine.

Goon PCP.

Goon Dust PCP.

Goosey Narcotics user considered untrustworthy.

Goric Paregoric.

Gorilla on (One's) Back Dependence on heroin requiring large doses to prevent withdrawal. From size of habit compared to "monkey," another term for narcotics dependency.

Gorilla Pills Barbiturates.

Gorilla Tab PCP.

Gosneaks Narcotics.

Got It Beat Past the most painful aspects of narcotics withdrawal.

Gouger Marihuana smoker.

Gow 1. Any narcotic. 2. Marihuana. 3. Opium.

Gow Cellar Place where narcotics are sold.

Gow Crust Opium ashes.

Gow Head Narcotics user.

Gowed Overdosed on narcotics.

Gowed Up Intoxicated by narcotics.

Gowster 1. Narcotics user. 2. Marihuana user.

Goynk Opium.

Grads Amphetamines.

Graduate To begin to use more potent drugs.

Grape Parfait LSD.

Grass Marihuana. The most popular term for marihuana in the 1960s, although the term originated much earlier.

Grass Action Buying marihuana.

Grass Brownies Cookies baked with marihuana. *Same as* Alice B. Toklas Brownies.

Grass Eater Marihuana user.

Grass Party Party at which marihuana is smoked.

Grass Pipe Pipe for smoking marihuana or hashish.

Grasshopper 1. Marihuana user. 2. Luggage for smuggling marihuana.

Gravy Mixture of heroin and blood in a syringe.

Grease Opium prepared for smoking.

Greasy Junkie Narcotics user who begs for money rather than trying to get it by other means.

Greefa, Greefo, Grefa, Grifa, Griffa, Grifo Marihuana.

Greefer Marihuana smoker.

Green 1. Marihuana. 2. Marihuana cigarette. 3. Ketamine hydrochloride. 4. PCP.

Green Ashes Opium ashes.

Green Dragon 1. Barbiturates. 2. Amphetamines. 3. LSD used in combination with belladonna alkaloids, e.g., belladonna, datura.

Green Griff Marihuana.

Green Hornet Combination of dextroamphetamines and amobarbital.

Green Hype Beginning narcotics user.

Green Moroccan Hashish from Morocco, green in color.

Green Mud Opium that has not been properly prepared for smoking.

Green Swirls LSD.

Green Tea PCP.

Green Wedge LSD.

Greenies Green tablets containing an amphetamine and a barbiturate.

Greens Marihuana.

Greese Opium.

Greese Pit Place where opium is sold.

Griefer Marihuana smoker.

Griefo Marihuana.

Grifado Intoxicated by marihuana.

Grocery Boy Narcotics user with an appetite for food.

Grog 1. Alcohol. 2. Narcotics.

Grog Merchant Narcotics seller.

Groove, In the Using drugs.

Grooving Feeling euphoric following drug use.

Ground Control, Controller *Same as* Babysitter.

Groundman *Same as* Babysitter.

G-shot 1. Small dose of heroin solution taken to ward off discomfort associated with narcotics withdrawal until larger amount can be obtained. 2. Small amount of heroin given to taste face for loan of his paraphernalia.

Gum Opium that is eaten.

Gumdrop 1. Seconal, a barbiturate. 2. Any drug in capsule form.

Gun Hypodermic needle.

Gun Powder Opium.

Gungeon, Gunja, Gunjeh 1. Marihuana. 2. Marihuana from Jamaica. 3. Term used during the 1940s for the most potent form of marihuana which sold for one dollar per cigarette.

Gunk 1. Morphine. 2. Inhalants.

Gunny Marihuana.

Gunny Dodger One who injects cocaine and morphine mixtures.

Gups Narcotics.

Guru 1. Guide or authority. 2. One who initiates someone else into drug use. 3. *Same as* Babysitter.

Gutter Vein (median cubital) in the crook of the elbow, a favorite site for narcotics injection.

Gyves Marihuana cigarette. Possibly a variant of Jive. (1930s).

H

H Heroin.

H and C Hot and cold. Mixture of heroin and cocaine.

H Caps Heroin in capsules.

Habit 1. Dependence on narcotics. 2. Craving for narcotics; a condition brought on by habitual usage.

Habit-forming Can produce dependence.

Habitual Chronic; on a regular basis.

Habituation Psychological, in contrast to physiological, dependence. A condition in which the user feels a desire, but not a compulsion, to continue drug use for a sense of well-being and feels discomfort when deprived of it. There is little tendency to increase the dosage in connection with habituation. The term has come into disuse because of the difficulty in distinguishing between it and dependence.

Had Taken advantage of.

Hag Narcotics user who needs a large amount of drug to prevent withdrawal.

Haidar, Cup of Hashish.

Haidar, Emerald Cup of Hashish.

Haight *See* Haight-Ashbury.

Haight-Ashbury Intersection of streets in San Francisco that became synonymous with the drug culture of the 1960s.

Hairy Heroin.

Half One-half ounce of adulterated, street-quality heroin. About fifteen five-dollar bags.

Half-bundle About twelve five-dollar bags of heroin.

Half-load About fifteen three-dollar bags of heroin.

Half-moon Bulk marihuana sold in the shape of a half-moon.

Half-piece One-half ounce of narcotics.

Half-spoon One-half gram of cocaine.

Halfway House Facility in which someone who has been discharged from a treatment center lives as he/she readjusts to living in society.

Hallucination Perception that has no external stimulus.

Hallucinogen Substance producing hallucinations, that is, perceptions unrelated to external stimuli, for example, LSD, peyote, psilocybin. From the Greek word *halucinari*, "to wander mentally." Generally refers to DMT, LSD, mescaline, peyote, psilocybin, and psilocin. Other drugs such as marihuana and alcohol may also produce hallucinations but are not classified as hallucinogens because these substances do not usually produce these effects.

Haloperidol Antipsychotic tranquilizer. Trade name is Haldol.

Halvahed Under the influence of heroin.

Halvah Heroin.

Hand to Hand Delivery of drugs personally to buyer rather than "dropping" or leaving them to be picked up.

Hang In To keep trying.

Hang Loose To relax; be calm.

Hang Tough To undergo withdrawal from narcotics abruptly and without help.

Hang Up 1. A bother, concern. 2. Abstention from drugs.

Hangout Place to gather, associate, congregate with others of similar temperament and interests.

Happening Any event.

Happy Cigarette Marihuana cigarette.

Happy Dust 1. Narcotics. 2. Cocaine.

Happy Flakes Narcotics in powder form.

Happy Gas Marihuana.

Happy Grass Marihuana.

Happy Medicine Morphine.

Happy Powder 1. Narcotics in powder form. 2. Cocaine.

Happy Stuff 1. Narcotics. 2. Cocaine.

Hard Drugs Drugs that produce physiological dependence.

Hard Nail Needle used for narcotics injection.

Hard Stuff Drugs that produce physiological dependence.

Hard Time Time spent in prison.

Hard Times Scarcity of drugs.

Hardware Brand name for amyl nitrite.

Harpoon Needle used for narcotics injection.

Harrison Narcotics Act U.S. antinarcotics law. The Harrison Act came into effect in 1915 and was the first such American law and the basis for all subsequent antidrug laws. It required dealers in narcotics to register with the Bureau of Internal Revenue and pay a small fee for a tax stamp. Narcotics users were not permitted to buy such stamps, so they could only get drugs from authorized dealers. The intent of the law was not initially punitive but rather to gain control over domestic drug sale, distribution, and usage. However, possession of narcotics soon became illegal under the law.

Harry Heroin.

Has Marihuana.

Hash Hashish.

Hash Cannon *See* Carburetor.

Hash Head Frequent user of hashish.

Hash Oil Distillate of marihuana or hashish, viscous and very potent. Marihuana is extracted in boiling alcohol, which dissolves cannabinoids. Noncannabinoids are strained off. The solvent is then evaporated, leaving concentrated oil containing 40 to 60 percent THC. The oil can be applied to tobacco cigarettes or to marihuana cigarettes to increase their potency. Appeared in the United States in 1970. *See* Son of One.

Hashbury *See* Haight-Ashbury.

Hashish The resin-covered flowers or bracts of cannabis which generally contain more THC than other parts of the plant. Considered to be more potent than marihuana, but this distinction is disappearing due to the higher-potency marihuana that is now available. In contrast to marihuana, which is sold as leaves and stems, hashish is sold in the form of soft or hard balls or tablets and, is smoked in pipes or cigarettes. Originally a general Arabic term for grass or fodder, medicinal herbs, or weeds. *Hashish* evolved as a nickname for the "herb"—cannabis. In India hashish is called *charas*.

Hashish Club *See* Club des Haschischins.

Hashish Oil *See* Hash Oil.

Hassle 1. Inconvenience; problem; unpleasant situation. 2. Difficulty in buying drugs. 3. Harassment by police.

Have a Habit To be dependent on drugs.

Have a Yen To crave drugs.

Have an Itch To crave drugs.

Have On the Feed Bag To be under the influence of narcotics.

Have You Got a Thing? Have you got any drugs to sell?

Hawaiian Sunshine 1. LSD. 2. Marihuana.

Hawk, the LSD.

Hay Marihuana.

Hay Burner Marihuana smoker.

Hay Butt Marihuana cigarette.

Hay Head Chronic marihuana smoker.

Haze LSD.

Hazel Heroin.

H-cap Capsule of heroin.

Head Chronic drug user. Someone who has made drug use an important part of his or her life.

Head and Body Trip Drug reaction that involves both physiological and psychological sensations.

Head Drug Drug affecting the mind, primarily through altering consciousness.

Head Gear Drug paraphernalia, for example, pipes, papers, clips.

Head Shop Store selling paraphernalia for drug use.

Headshrinker Psychiatrist or psychologist.

Heaped Under the influence of drugs.

Heart On Brand name for amyl nitrite.

Hearts Amphetamines, usually Dexedrine or Benzedrine.

Heat 1. Police. 2. Harassment by police.

Heat's On Police are looking for drug users to arrest.

Heaven and Hell PCP.

Heaven Dust Cocaine.

Heavenly Blues 1. LSD. 2. Morning-glory seeds.

Heavenly Sunshine LSD.

Heaves Vomiting resulting from alcohol-induced gastritis, withdrawal from narcotics, or response to a hitherto naive user's first injection of heroin.

Heaves and Squirts Vomiting and diarrhea. *See* Heaves.

Heavy 1. Profound; considerable. 2. Potent.

Heavy Drugs Narcotics.

Heavy Hash Potent hashish.

Heavy Joint Marihuana cigarette to which PCP has been added.

Heavy Man Drug seller.

Heavy Stuff Drugs that produce physiological dependence.

Hedonistic Pleasure-seeking. Often used in reference to drug users and their motivation for drug use.

Heel Tap Chloral hydrate.

Heeled 1. Having money. 2. Carrying a gun.

Heesh Hashish.

Hell Dust 1. Heroin. 2. Morphine.

Helen Heroin.

Hemp 1. The bast fiber of the marihuana plant, *Cannabis sativa*. 2. General term for many different bast fibers, for example, jute, sisal. 3. Marihuana.

Henry Heroin.

Hep 1. Aware; knowledgeable. 2. Sophisticated.

Hepatitis Inflammation of the liver, disorder sometimes related to use of contaminated needles by narcotics users.

Heptabarbital Short-acting barbiturate.

Her Cocaine.

Herb Marihuana.

Herms PCP.

Hero Heroin.

Heroin Semisynthetic derivative of morphine. Chemical name is diacetylmorphine hydrochloride. Synthesized in 1898 in Germany. Name is derived from the German word *heroisch*, meaning "heroic; powerful." Comes in the form of a powder or tablet.

Heroin Buzz Most-potent form of PCP, brown in color.

Heroin maintenance Legal administration of heroin by prescription, used primarily in England. In the United States methadone maintenance is the rule.

Heroin No. 3 Low-potency, granular, light brown heroin mixture to which caffeine and other ingredients have been added. Manufactured in Hong Kong and sold primarily to Asian users. Contains about 20 to 30 percent pure heroin.

Heroin No. 4 High-potency, fluffy, white powdered heroin manufactured in Hong Kong. Very soluble in water. Contains about 80 to 95 percent pure heroin. Used in United States and Europe.

Hexobarbital Short-acting barbiturate.

Hi Baller Brand name for amyl nitrite.

Hide the Flag To cover up the odor of opium by pouring oil of wintergreen onto newspapers and warming them so that fumes will be given off.

High 1. Drunk. 2. Intoxicated by psychoactive drugs. The term most frequently used to describe the pleasurable effects of marihuana. 3. Euphoric; exhilarated.

High and Light Mildly intoxicated by a drug.

High as a Kite Intoxicated by a drug.

High Fi Mixture of morphine and cocaine.

High Hat 1. Large bolus of opium. 2. Stage of narcotics usage in which a large amount of drug is needed to prevent withdrawal.

High Stepper Narcotics user who buys his drugs in the better part of a city.

Higher Than a Kite *Same as* High as a Kite.

Highsiding *Same as* High.

Hikori, Hikuli Peyote.

Him Heroin.

Himmelsbach test Test for assessing the severity of withdrawal from narcotics by assigning points to various symptoms.

Hip 1. Aware; knowledgeable. 2. Sophisticated.

Hippies Individuals following a way of life based on renunciation of material things and believing it possible to achieve deep insight into life through use of drugs. Hippies flourished during the 1960s and early 1970s. *See also* Counterculture.

Histadyl Antihistamine that contains codeine.

Hit 1. To purchase drugs. 2. To dilute a drug. 3. To smoke marihuana, swallow drugs, or inject narcotics intravenously. 4. To take a deep inhalation from a marihuana cigarette. 5. Intense reaction from narcotics. 6. Assassination.

Hit and Miss Habit *Same as* Chipping.

Hit by the Hop Dependent on opium.

Hit Spike Improvised needle for narcotics injection.

Hit the Gong To smoke opium in the company of others.

Hit the Gow 1. To use narcotics. 2. Dependent on narcotics.

Hit the Hay To smoke marihuana.

Hit the Hop To use opium.

Hit the Moon To become very intoxicated by a drug.

Hit the Pipe To smoke opium.

Hit the Sewer To inject narcotics intravenously.

Hit the Stem To smoke opium.

Hit the Stuff To use narcotics.

Hitch Up the Reindeer To arrange the paraphernalia for using cocaine.

Hits Combination of codeine and Doriden.

H.M.C. Mixture of heroin, morphine, and cocaine.

Hobster Narcotics user.

Hocus, Hokus Morphine, heroin, or cocaine in solution.

HOG 1. Hash, O, Grass. Term for marihuana used by American soldiers in Vietnam. 2. Narcotics user who requires large doses to prevent withdrawal. 3. PCP.

Hold Your High To maintain ability to function normally while under the influence of drugs.

Holding Possessing drugs.

Holistic treatment Method of treating drug abuse that goes beyond dealing with the specific problem and involves a total change in life-style.

Home 1. Vein (median cubital) in the crook of the elbow, a favorite site for narcotics injection. 2. The solvent used to prepare cocaine freebase. From metaphor of cocaine freebase and baseball. *See* Baseball; First Baseman.

Homegrown Domestic marihuana; marihuana grown in someone's home or backyard.

Honey Oil Hashish oil.

Honeymoon Initial period of narcotics usage during which small doses are taken.

Hooch, Hootch Marihuana.

Hookah Water pipe for smoking marihuana, hashish, tobacco, and so on. Smoke is first drawn through water and cooled, making it less harsh.

Hooked Dependent on drugs, usually used in reference to narcotics.

Hoosier, Hoosier Fiend 1. Naive user of narcotics. 2. Narcotics user who has not recognized that he has become dependent.

Hop 1. Opium. 2. Narcotics. 3. Any drug of abuse.

Hop Fiend Narcotics or marihuana user.

Hop Gun Hypodermic syringe.

Hop Head, Hophead Narcotics or marihuana user. Originally an opium user.

Hop Hog *Same as* Hop Head.

Hop Joint Place where opium is smoked.

Hop Layout Paraphernalia for smoking opium.

Hop Merchant Narcotics seller.

Hop on the Monkey Wagon To become dependent on narcotics.

Hop Party 1. Party at which opium is smoked. 2. Party at which marihuana is smoked.

Hop Simple Opium user who doesn't know very much about the drug.

Hop Stick Pipe for smoking opium.

Hop Toy Small container of opium.

Hopped, Hopped Up Under the influence of narcotics.

Hopper Narcotics user. Originally an opium user.

Hoppie Narcotics user.

Hoppy Dust Cocaine.

Hops Dried flowers of the hop plant, used to flavor beer.

Hops Stick Opium pipe.

Hops Stiff *Same as* Hopper.

Hopster *Same as* Hopper.

Horn 1. To sniff cocaine. 2. To sniff heroin.

Horner Cocaine user.

Horror Drug Combination of LSD and datura.

Horrors 1. Delirium tremens. 2. Paranoia concerning arrest for drug possession.

Hors d'oeuvres 1. Seconal. 2. Any drug in capsule form.

Horse Heroin.

Horse and Wagon Hypodermic needle and syringe.

Horse Heads Amphetamines.

Horse Radish Heroin.

Horse Trank PCP.

Horse Tranquilizer PCP.

Horsed Under the influence of heroin.

Hospital Heroin Dilaudid.

Hot Bag Dead body containing evidence of polydrug use.

Hot Box Room filled with marihuana smoke.

Hot Dream Dream experienced while under the influence of opium.

Hot Hay Marihuana.

Hot Shot Dose of heroin that is fatal due to the presence of a contaminant such as cyanide.

Hot Stick Marihuana cigarette.

Hot Stuff Counterfeit or low-potency narcotics.

How Much Are You Holding? 1. How much money do you have to contribute toward purchase of a group bottle? 2. What is the quantity of drugs in your possession?

HRN Heroin.

Hubble-Bubble Water-cooled pipe. *See* Hookah.

Huffer Glue or gasoline sniffer.

Hummer An arrest for a minor infraction, enabling police to search for drugs.

Humming Gay Opium pipe bowl that sizzles while opium is cooking.

Humming Gee Bowl Pipe for smoking opium. The bowl has the shape of a skull.

Humping the Sage Smoking marihuana.

Hung Out, Hung Up 1. Dependent on drugs. 2. Bothered by problems.

Hungries Craving for food after smoking marihuana.

Hungry Horrors Craving for food following withdrawal from alcohol or other drugs.

Hunk Quarter-ounce or more of hashish.

Hurting 1. In need of narcotics to prevent withdrawal. 2. Experiencing the early feelings of withdrawal from narcotics.

Hustle To be involved with various activities to raise money to buy drugs.

Hydrocarbons Organic compounds, some of which are inhaled for their intoxicating effects.

Hydromorphone hydrochloride Chemical name for the narcotic Dilaudid.

Hyoscine Scopolamine.

Hyoscyamine Psychoactive ingredient in many plants that cause hallucinations, for example, jimson weed, datura, belladonna.

Hype Narcotics user who administers his drug intravenously. From *hypodermic*.

Hype Shooter *See* Hype.

Hype Shot Intravenous injection of narcotics.

Hype Stick Hypodermic syringe.

Hyped Under the influence of a narcotic.

Hypnotics Drugs causing sleep and confusion.

Hypo Juggler *See* Hype.

Hypo Smacker, Smecker *See* Hype. From *hypodermic* and *Schmeck*, a term for heroin.

I

Ice Cocaine.

Ice Bag Potent marihuana allegedly smuggled into California inside boxes of frozen lettuce.

Ice Cream Opium.

Ice Cream Habit Intermittent use of narcotics. *Same as* Chipping.

Ice Cream Man Opium seller.

Ice Pack *Same as* Ice Bag.

Ice Tong Doctor Physician who sells narcotics.

Ice Water Cure *Same as* Cold Turkey.

Ice Water John Physician who does not provide drugs to ease narcotics withdrawal.

Iced In jail.

Ickey 1. In need of narcotics to prevent withdrawal. 2. Hypodermic needle.

Idiot Juice Mixture of nutmeg and water.

Idiot Pills 1. Barbiturates. 2. Doriden.

Illicit Drug Drug whose manufacture, sale, or use is prohibited by law.

Illusion Distortion in perception of a stimulus; in contrast to a hallucination, which has no basis in external stimulation.

I'm Looking Who can I buy drugs from?

Imipramine hydrochloride Antidepressant. Trade name is Tofranil.

Importer First receiver of heroin in United States. Major figure in bringing drug into country. Sells drug to kilo connection.

Impotence Decrease in or absence of the ability in males to function sexually; or decrease in or absence of fertility.

In Under the influence of a psychoactive drug.

In a Nod Under the influence of a drug.

In Dreams Using opium.

In Flight Intoxicated by amphetamines.

In Front of the Gun Selling drugs with the understanding that the seller will not reveal his source.

In Orbit *Same as* In Flight.

In Paper Narcotics concealed in or under paper, such as postage stamps, which are smuggled into prison.

In the Air Intoxicated by marihuana.

In the Business Using narcotics.

In the Chips Using narcotics irregularly.

In Transit Under the influence of LSD.

In Trouble Experiencing the early effects of withdrawal from narcotics.

In Tweeds Using marihuana.

In vitro Outside the body. Generally refers to chemical reactions occurring in test tubes, flasks, etc.

In vivo Inside the body. Generally refers to chemical reactions occurring in the body.

Inbetweens 1. Amphetamines. 2. Barbiturates.

Incense Marihuana.

Incentive Cocaine.

Indian Bay Marihuana.

Indian Hay Marihuana.

Indian Hemp Marihuana.

Indian Hemp Drugs Commission First government-sponsored study of the physical, mental, and moral effects of marihuana. Conducted 1893–1894 in India. The report filled seven volumes totaling 3,281 pages.

Indian Oil Hashish Oil.

Indian Rope Potent hashish from India.

Indian Weed Marihuana.

Indications Medical conditions for which drug use is recognized.

Inger To feign withdrawal in hopes of convincing a physician to administer or prescribe narcotics.

Inhalant Organic solvent inhaled for its psychoactive effect, for example, glue, polish remover.

Inner Itch Craving for narcotics.

Instant Zen LSD.

Institutionalized Placed in a clinic or other center for prolonged treatment of an alcohol- or drug-related problem.

Interaction Intensification or diminution of a drug's effects by another drug.

Into 1. Using drugs. 2. Concerned or involved with something.

Intoxed Intoxicated by alcohol or some other psychoactive substance. *See* Intoxication.

Intoxication Altered state of consciousness caused by alcohol or other psychoactive substances which results in a diminished capacity to function.

Isobutyl nitrite Vasodilator used as a stimulant. Considered to have aphrodisiaclike effects.

Isonipecaine Meperidine.

Iron Cure *Same as* Ice Water Cure.

Iron House Jail.

Isda Heroin.

Isomer Compound with the same composition and molecular weight as another compound, but with different chemical properties.

Isomerize To rearrange atoms in a molecule so that physical and chemical properties are changed, although molecular weight remains the same, for example, cannabidiol to tetrahydrocannabinol.

Isomerizer Drug paraphernalia device for changing other cannabinoids into tetrahydrocannabinol, thereby increasing the potency of marihuana.

J

J (Jay) Marihuana cigarette. *Abbreviation of* Joint.

J (Jay) Pipe Pipe for smoking marihuana.

J (Jay) Smoke Marihuana.

Jab Injection of narcotics.

Jab Artist Narcotics user who is very adept at intravenous injections.

Jab Pop Intravenous injection of narcotics.

Jabber Narcotics user who injects his or her drug.

Jac Aroma Brand name for amyl nitrite.

Jack, Jack Off 1. *Same as* Boot. 2. To masturbate.

Jack Up Amytal Sodium.

Jackal To buy drugs as a means of gathering evidence of such for law enforcement purposes.

Jacked Up Under the influence of a psychoactive drug.

Jacking Off the Spike *Same as* Jack, Jack Off.

Jag 1. Under the influence of a drug. 2. Uncontrollable behavior, for example, a "laughing jag" from smoking marihuana.

Jahooby Marihuana.

Jail Plant Drugs smuggled into jail by a visitor.

Jailhouse High Euphoria from inhaling nutmeg or mace.

Jaloney Low-potency or counterfeit narcotics.

Jam 1. Amphetamines. 2. Cocaine. 3. Drug overdose. 4. Trouble.

Jam Cecil Amphetamines.

Jamaican Potent marihuana from Jamaica.

Jammed Taken an overdose.

Jane Marihuana.

Jane's Better Half Marihuana user.

J.C.L. Johnny-come-lately. A novice user of narcotics; one who has not yet developed a dependence.

Jee Gee Heroin.

Jefferson Airplane Device used to hold a burning marihuana cigarette butt.

Jelly Babies Amphetamines.

Jelly Beans 1. Amphetamines. 2. Any drug in capsule form.

Jenny Barn Women's area of a hospital housing narcotics users.

Jerk Off *Same as* Jack, Jack Off.

Jersey Green Domestic marihuana grown in New Jersey.

Jet Ketamine.

Jet Fuel PCP.

Jimson weed *Datura stramonium.* Weed containing alkaloids such as atropine, scopolamine, that can produce hallucinations.

Jingo Marihuana.

Jive 1. Marihuana. 2. Insincerity.

Jive Do Jee Heroin.

Jive Sticks Marihuana cigarettes.

Job's Antidote Hypodermic syringe.

Jockey Narcotics dependence.

Jocular 1. Drunk. 2. Intoxicated by marihuana.

John 1. Someone who does not use drugs. 2. Someone who patronizes prostitutes.

Johnson Marihuana.

Johnson and Johnson Hypodermic syringe.

Joint 1. Hand-rolled marihuana cigarette. 2. Paraphernalia for narcotics injection. 3. Opium den. 4. Bar or tavern. 5. Place to live. 6. Jail. 7. Penis.

Jojee Heroin.

Jolly Beans Amphetamines.

Jolly Pop Heroin injected irregularly.

Jolt Initial effect of alcohol, marihuana, or other psychoactive drug.

Jones 1. Heroin. 2. Dependence on narcotics. 3. Marihuana cigarette.

Joy Marihuana.

Joy Dust 1. Morphine. 2. Heroin. 3. Cocaine.

Joy Flakes 1. Morphine. 2. Heroin. 3. Cocaine.

Joy Juice Chloral hydrate.

Joy Pellet Capsule of amphetamines or barbiturates.

Joy Pop Injection of narcotics into muscles or under skin.

Joy Popper Irregular user of narcotics. *Same as* Chipper.

Joy Powder 1. Cocaine. 2. Heroin. 3. Morphine.

Joy Prick Narcotics injection.

Joy Ride Euphoric sensation resulting from drug or alcohol use.

Joy Rider Irregular user of drugs.

Joy Smoke Marihuana.

Joy Stick 1. Marihuana cigarette. 2. Opium pipe.

Ju Ju, Juju Marihuana.

Juan Valdez Marihuana.

Juana Marihuana.

Juane Marihuana.

Juanita Marihuana.

Juanita Weed Marihuana.

Judas Minerva *Same as* Jackal.

Jug 1. Large bottle of alcohol. 2. Vial of methadone. 3. Vial of methamphetamine.

Juggle To sell heroin.

Juggler Heroin dealer who buys from street dealer and sells to street addict.

Jugs Amphetamines.

Juice 1. Dilaudid. 2. PCP.

Junk Narcotics, usually heroin.

Junk Graft Narcotics traffic.

Junk Hog 1. Narcotics user. 2. Narcotics user who takes more drug than he needs or who takes drugs more often than he needs.

Junk Hound Narcotics addict.

Junk Man Narcotics user.

Junk Peddler Narcotics seller.

Junk Tank Jail cell in which drug addicts are held.

Junked, Junked Up Under the influence of narcotics.

Junker 1. Narcotics user. 2. Narcotics seller.

Junkerman Marihuana smoker.

Junkie 1. Someone dependent on narcotics. 2. Narcotics user who also sells narcotics.

K

K 1. Ketamine. 2. PCP, from its misrepresentation as ketamine.

Ka Ka 1. Heroin. 2. Low-potency or counterfeit heroin.

Kabayo Heroin.

Kaif, Keef, Kheef, Kif 1. Marihuana. 2. Hashish.

Kanjac Marihuana. Term used in Panama Canal Zone during the 1920s.

Kaps PCP.

K-blast PCP.

Kee, Key, Ki Kilogram (2.2 pounds).

Keef *See* Kaif, Keef, Kheef, Kif.

Keek Narcotics user who injects his drug.

Keeler Chloral hydrate.

Keep Off the Grass Don't use marihuana.

Keep the Meet To meet a drug seller at an agreed upon place and time.

Keester Plant Concealment of drugs in the rectum, usually by placing them in a condom or other container first. Used in prisons.

Keg Kilogram.

Keg Party Party where alcohol is consumed.

Kenkoy Heroin.

Ketamine 1. General anesthetic that causes hallucinations. 2. Misnomer for PCP.

Keyed, Keyed Up 1. Intoxicated by marihuana. 2. Nervous; distraught.

Keyster Plant *Same as* Keester Plant.

Khat Leaves of *Catha edulins*, a plant indigenous to the Middle East. Has a stimulant effect.

Khutchu String Marihuana.

Kick 1. Excitement; reaction; euphoric sensation; elation from drug use. 2. To give up drug use.

Kick Back To return to narcotics use after becoming detoxified.

Kick Cold Abrupt withdrawal from narcotics in contrast to gradual, drug-assisted withdrawal.

Kick Freak Irregular narcotics user; one who wishes to experience the sensations of drug use without becoming dependent.

Kick Stick Marihuana cigarette.

Kick the Clouds Under the influence of narcotics.

Kick the Gong To smoke opium.

Kick the Habit To stop using narcotics.

Kick the Pipe Around To smoke opium.

Kick the Rag To smoke opium.

Kick the Tip *Same as* Kick the Habit.

Kick the Toy To smoke opium.

Kicked by a Horse Dependent on heroin.

Kicked Up Intoxicated by narcotics.

Kicking It Out Trying to give up using narcotics.

Kidstuff Marihuana.

Kiester Plant *Same as* Keester Plant.

Kiester Stash *Same as* Keester Plant.

Kif *See* Kaif, Keef, Kheef, Kif.

Killer, Killer Stick Marihuana cigarette.

Killer Weed 1. Marihuana. 2. Marihuana mixed with PCP. 3. PCP.

Kilo Connection Second major distributor of heroin. Buys from importer, dilutes it by half, and sells to connection.

Kilter Marihuana.

King Kong Heavy dependence on narcotics; large monkey on one's back.

King Kong Pills 1. Barbiturates. 2. Doriden.

King Kongs *Same as* King Kong Pills.

Kipping Sleeping after having undergone narcotics withdrawal.

Kiss To blow exhaled cocaine freebase into someone's mouth.

Kiss Mary Jane To smoke marihuana.

Kit Paraphernalia for intravenous injection. *Same as* Artillery.

Kitchen Lab Illegal-drug-producing laboratory.

Kite Ounce of marihuana.

K.J. Krystal Joint, marihuana to which PCP has been added.

K.J. Crystal *Same as* K.J.

Knife in the Arm Crude injection of narcotics.

Knock Yourself Crazy To smoke marihuana.

Knocked Out Under the influence of narcotics.

Knocker Someone opposed to drug use.

Knocking on the Door Trying to stay away from other narcotics users.

Knockout Drops Drug given to produce unconsciousness. Usually refers to chloral hydrate mixed with alcohol.

Kokomo Cocaine user.

Kokomo Joe *Same as* Kokomo.

Kona Gold Potent marihuana from the Hawaiian island of Kona.

Kona Kona *Same as* Kona Gold.

Konk, Konk Out To become unconscious due to narcotics overdose.

Kook *Same as* Keek.

Kools PCP.

K.O.'s Opium.

Krystal Joint Marihuana to which PCP has been added.

KW PCP.

L

L LSD.

La Guardia Report (The Marihuana Problem in the City of New York) First detailed sociological and clinical study of the effects of marihuana. The report was initiated by the New York Academy of Medicine in 1938 at the request of New York Mayor Fiorello La Guardia. The study was conducted between 1940 and 1941. The report was published in 1944.

L.A. Turnabouts Amphetamines.

LAAM Levo-alpha-acetylmethadol, a long-acting narcotic antagonist used in maintenance programs.

Lability Instability.

Laced Alcohol or drug added to another drug or beverage.

Lactose Milk sugar, an inert material used to dilute other drugs to increase their bulk.

Lady Cocaine.

Lady Snow Cocaine.

Lady White 1. Cocaine. 2. Narcotics in powder form.

Laid Out Under the influence of marihuana.

Lame 1. Someone who doesn't smoke marihuana. 2. Naive narcotics user. 3. Weak; feeble.

Lame Duck Nonuser of narcotics.

Lamp Habit Dependent on opium.

Laodicean Beginning narcotics user. Reference to city of Laodicea where early Christians were not very devout.

Lard Police officer.

Laudanum Alcoholic solution containing 10 percent opium. Used primarily during the nineteenth century. From the Latin *ladanum*, a yellow resin.

Laugh and Scratch 1. Intravenous narcotics use. 2. Marihuana use.

Laughing Gas Nitrous oxide.

Laughing Grass Marihuana.

Laughing Jag Uncontrollable laughter.

Laughing Tobacco Marihuana.

Laughing Weed Marihuana.

Launch Pad Place where drugs are taken by a group.

Lay 1. To sell marihuana or offer it as an unsolicited gift. 2. To smoke opium. 3. Place where opium is smoked.

Lay against the Engine To smoke opium.

Lay Down 1. To smoke opium. 2. Cost of entry into an opium den.

Lay Down Joint, Lay Joint Place where opium is smoked.

Lay the Stem To smoke opium.

Layette Paraphernalia for smoking opium.

Laying Down the Hustle Selling marihuana or other drugs.

Laying on the Hip Smoking opium. From the position adopted in opium dens when smoking the drug.

Laying the Hypo Injecting narcotics.

Layout Paraphernalia for smoking opium or injecting other narcotics.

LBJ 1. Heroin. 2. LSD. 3. Mixture of LSD, barbiturates, and heroin. 4. Piperydil benzilate hydrochloride, a hallucinogen.

Leaf Narcotics, usually opium.

Leaf Gum Crude opium.

Leaf Hop *Same as* Leaf Gum.

Lean against the Engine To smoke opium.

Leaner Destitute person who does not have money for even the poorest accommodations.

Leapers 1. Amphetamines. 2. Heavy users of cocaine.

Leaping and Stinking Under the influence of narcotics or cocaine.

Leaps Uncontrollable excitement and movement resulting from excessive use of cocaine.

Leather Dew Low-potency narcotics.

Leaves Marihuana.

Leb, Lebanese Hashish from Lebanon.

LeDain Commission *See* Canadian Commission of Inquiry into the Nonmedical Use of Drugs.

Leepers *Same as* Leapers.

Legal high Euphoria from use of various herbs, spices, and chemicals that can be legally obtained, such as nutmeg, catnip, and wild lettuce.

LEMAR First (1965) organized effort to work for legalization of marihuana.

Lem-kee Opium.

Lemmon 714 Methaqualone. 714 derives from number scored on 300-milligram tablet manufactured by Lemmon Pharmaceuticals under brand name of Quaalude.

Lemmons Methaqualone, from the name of Lemmon Pharmaceuticals, which manufactures drug.

Lemon Low-potency or counterfeit drugs.

Lemon Bowl Lemon rind placed inside bowl of an opium pipe to make the opium milder.

Lemonade 1. Weak marihuana. 2. Excessively diluted heroin.

Leno Marihuana cigarette.

Lenos PCP.

Lent Morphine.

Leper Grass Potent marihuana from Colombia.

Let It All Hang Out Hide nothing; be honest.

Let Me Go Give me some drugs.

Let Me Hold Something Do you have any drugs for sale?

Lettuce Money.

Lettuce Opium Wild lettuce (*Lacturca virosa*), which produces mild psychoactive effect similar to opium.

Levallorphan Tartrate Narcotic antagonist.

Levo-alpha-acetylmethadol *See* LAAM.

Levorphanol Tartrate Narcotic. Trade name is Levo-Dromoran.

Lhesca Marihuana.

Li Un Superior-quality opium.

Li Yuen Superior-quality opium.

Liability Risk of producing dependence.

Librium Trade name for chlordiazepoxide hydrochloride, an anti-anxiety tranquilizer.

Lick To ingest a drug.

Lid Small, clear plastic bag containing 1 to 2 ounces of loose, uncleaned marihuana. The bag is wrapped in thick roll and sealed with masking or Scotch tape. One lid will make about forty marihuana cigarettes.

Lid Action Purchase of a lid of marihuana.

Lid Poppers Amphetamines.

Lidocaine A local anesthetic.

Lie in State with the Girls To smoke marihuana. From the names Mary, Jane, Mary Warner, and such given to marihuana.

Lie on Your Hip To smoke opium.

Lift 1. Sensation from drug use. 2. Progression to stronger drugs.

Light Artillery Hypodermic syringe.

Light Green Marihuana.

Light Stuff Drugs that do not produce physical dependence.

Light Up To smoke marihuana.

Lightning Amphetamines.

Lightning Hashish Potent hashish used by dealers for their own personal enjoyment.

Lightning Smoke Adulterated opium.

Light-weight Chipper Irregular narcotics user.

Light-weight Nothing Irregular narcotics habit.

Lilly 1. Seconal. From the name of the drug company that manufactures it.

Lincoln Five-dollar bill.

Line 1. Vein into which narcotics are injected. *Abbreviation of* Mainline. 2. Narcotics injection. 3. Powdered drug formed into a line so that it can be sniffed through a straw.

Line Shot Intravenous injection of narcotics.

Liner Narcotics user who injects his drugs intravenously.

Lip the Dripper To make sure there is no air in the medicine dropper prior to intravenous injection.

Lipton's Weak marihuana (1940s).

Liquid Grass THC, tetrahydrocannabinol.

Liquid Hash Hashish oil.

Lit Up Under the influence of a drug, usually narcotics or marihuana.

Little D Dilaudid.

Live Bait Teenage drug users who sell drugs to other teenagers.

Live in the Suburbs To use narcotics sporadically.

Live Ones PCP.

L.L. Marihuana.

Load 1. Dose of narcotics. 2. Twenty-five bags of heroin.

Loaded Intoxicated by a drug.

Loaded on Back Intoxicated by a drug to the point of wanting to do nothing but rest.

Loads Codeine used in combination with Doriden.

Lob Loafer in an opium den.

Lobby Gow Loafer in an opium den.

Lobby Lob *Same as* Lobby Gow.

Lobo Marihuana.

Loc-A-Roma Brand name for amyl nitrite.

Locker Popper Brand name for amyl nitrite.

Locker Room Brand name for butyl nitrite.

Loco Weed Marihuana. Not to be confused with plant (*Astrafulus mollisimus*) also known as loco weed that makes cattle sick.

Locus Narcotics.

Locust Narcotics user.

Locust Point Distribution place where narcotics are sold to dealers.

Log 1. Marihuana cigarette. 2. Opium pipe.

Log Stick Opium pipe.

Long Tightly packed marihuana.

Long Run Extended period since last drug use resulting in initial feeling of withdrawal.

Longing Wanting drugs.

Long-tail Rat Drug user who informs on other drug users.

Look-Alikes Counterfeit drugs.

Looking *Same as* Longing.

Loose Relaxed.

Lords Dilaudid.

Lorfan Levallorphan tartrate.

Lose Your Cookies To vomit after drug use.

Louse Drug user who informs on other drug users.

Loused Covered with abscesses from intravenous injection of drugs.

Love Affair Mixture of cocaine and heroin.

Love Drug MDA.

Love Saves LSD solution on paper.

Love Weed Marihuana. From marihuana's alleged aphrodisiac properties.

Love Wood Hashish.

Lovely Combination of PCP and marihuana.

Lover Marihuana smoker.

Low Rider Destitute narcotics user.

Lozies Marihuana.

LSD Lysergic acid diethylamide–25, a hallucinogenic synthesized in 1938. Produced from lysergic acid, a substance derived from the ergot fungus that grows on rye, or from lysergic acid amide, an ingredient in morning-glory seeds. Psychoactive effects were discovered in 1943. Sold in tablet form, in squares of gelatin called windowpanes, on impregnated paper called blotter acid, or as a white, odorless powder. Effects are called a trip and last two to twelve hours and consist of altered perception, mood, and motor coordination. Unpleasant reactions include panic, anxiety, and confusion. Classified under Schedule 1 of the Controlled Substances Act.

Lucy in the Sky with Diamonds LSD.

Lude *Abbreviation for* Quaalude, a trade name for methaqualone, an antianxiety tranquilizer.

Luding Out Taking methaqualone.

Luer Glass syringe.

Lumber Stems of the marihuana plant.

Luminal Trade name for phenobarbital, a long-acting barbiturate.

Lusher Alcoholic who mixes marihuana with alcohol.

Lysergic Acid Amide Precursor of LSD. Found in some varieties of morning-glory seeds.

Lysergic Acid Diethylamide LSD.

M

M Refers to any drug whose name begins with this letter, for example, marihuana, morphine.

M and C Mixture of morphine and cocaine.

M and M's 1. Seconal capsules, a barbiturate. 2. Any drug in capsule form.

Mace Spice derived from nutmeg that has some hallucinogenic action due to mysticin.

Mach Marihuana.

Machine Needle used for intravenous injection.

Machinery 1. Paraphernalia for intravenous injection. *Same as* Artillery. 2. Marihuana.

Machu Picchu Potent marihuana from Peru.

Macoha Marihuana.

Macon Marihuana.

Maconha Marihuana.

Maggie Marihuana.

Magic PCP.

Magic Dust PCP.

Magic Mist PCP.

Magic Mushroom Psilocybin.

Magic Pumpkin Mescaline.

Maharishee Marihuana.

Mahoska Narcotics.

Main, Mainline 1. To inject a drug intravenously. 2. The vein (median cubital) in the crook of the elbow, a favorite site for narcotics injection.

Mainline Shooter *Same as* Mainliner.

Mainliner Drug user who injects his drug intravenously. Usually used in reference to narcotics.

Maintaining Keeping oneself at a particular level of drug use without affecting ability to function.

Maintenance therapy Treatment of drug dependence, usually narcotic dependence, by supplying that drug or one which will prevent withdrawal, for example, methadone, thereby permitting normal functioning.

Major tranquilizer Antipsychotic tranquilizer.

Majoun Marihuana.

Make To identify someone as a drug seller or a narcotics officer.

Make a Buy To purchase drugs.

Make a Croaker for a Reader To feign withdrawal in hopes of convincing a physician to administer or prescribe narcotics.

Make a Spread To lay out the paraphernalia for narcotics injection.

Make It Steel and Concrete To undergo withdrawal from narcotics without the help of drugs.

Make Pay Dirt To buy drugs.

Make the Drive To smuggle drugs into prison.

Make the Man To buy drugs.

Make Tracks To leave suddenly.

Make Your Nose Itch To sniff powdered narcotics.

Man, the 1. Police officer. 2. Seller of drugs.

Man from Montana Marihuana seller.

Mandragora Mandrake.

Mandrax British manufactured drug containing methaqualone and diphenhydramine, an antihistamine.

Manhattan Silver Light-colored marihuana allegedly grown in sewers of New York as a result of being flushed down the toilet to avoid arrest for possession. Considered to be very potent. Silver color is allegedly due to growth in absence of sun, preventing photosynthesis.

Manhattan White *Same as* Manhattan Silver.

Mahogany Juice Opium.

Manicure To remove stems and seeds from crude marihuana.

Manicured Cleaned marihuana.

Manita Milk sugar used to dilute heroin.

MAO inhibitor Monoamine oxidase inhibitor, a class of antidepressant drugs.

Marathon Encounter Lengthy group-therapy session.

Marathons Amphetamines.

Marc Residue remaining on the cotton after heroin has been filtered through it.

Marfil Brand of marihuana cigarette paper.

Margin Man Middleman in the sale of narcotics, usually the one who distributes to the local seller.

Mari, Mary Marihuana.

Mariahuana Marihuana.

Mariguana Marihuana.

Marihuana Mixture of leaves, flowers, and stems from the plant *Cannabis sativa* or *Cannabis indica*. It has the potential for intoxication due to its content of delta–9-tetrahydrocannabinol. The etymology of the word is unknown. It most likely derived from the Mexican-Spanish *mariguana*, meaning "intoxicant."

Marihuana and Health Reporting Act of 1970 Law requiring the Secretary of Health, Education, and Welfare to report annually concerning current information on the health consequences of marihuana.

Marihuana Tax Act of 1937 Federal antimarihuana law requiring anyone buying marihuana to obtain a tax stamp.

Marijuana Marihuana.

Mariweegee Marihuana.

Marmon Morphine.

Marmon and Cadillac Combination of morphine and cocaine.

Marshmallow Reds Red capsules of Seconal, a barbiturate.

Mary 1. Morphine. 2. Marihuana.

Mary and Johnny Marihuana.

Mary Ann Marihuana.

Mary Anner Marihuana.

Mary Jane Marihuana.

Mary Jane Cigarettes Marihuana cigarettes.

Mary Juana Marihuana.

Mary Owsley Solution of LSD.

Mary Warmer Marihuana.

Mary Warner Marihuana.

Mary Weaver Marihuana.

Mary Werner Marihuana.

Mary Worner Marihuana.

Master Key Sledgehammer used by police to break down a door.

Match *Abbreviation for* Matchbox.

Matchbox About one-fifth of a lid. It makes up to five to ten marihuana cigarettes.

Matchhead Quantity of PCP (about 8 milligrams) the size of a matchhead. Sold for about two dollars in 1980.

Matsakaw Heroin.

Maude C Narcotics.

Maui (Wowie) Potent marihuana from Hawaiian island of Maui.

Mayo 1. Cocaine. 2. Heroin. 3. Morphine.

Mayor's Committee on Marihuana *See* La Guardia Report (The Marihuana Problem in the City of New York).

McCoy Relatively pure narcotics.

MDA Methylenedioxyamphetamine. Drug is similar in structure to amphetamines and mescaline. Present in nutmeg.

MDB Pemoline.

Mean Very good.

Mean Green PCP.

Meat Wagon Ambulance.

MED Codeine.

Medical drug use In contrast to nonmedical drug use, use of drugs for sanctioned medical purposes.

Medicine Methadone.

Meet Meeting between drug buyer and drug seller.

Megg Marihuana.

Mellow 1. Pleasant; enjoyable. 2. Calm; relaxed.

Mellow Drug of America MDA.

Mellow Dude Calm individual who is able to control his emotions.

Mellow Yellow 1. 1960s hoax. Inside scrapings from banana skins that were baked, then smoked, allegedly producing effects akin to marihuana. The hoax originated in Haight-Ashbury and was disseminated by the underground press. 2. LSD.

Melt Wax To smoke opium.

Melter Morphine.

Meperidine hydrochloride Synthetic narcotic used as an analgesic, especially in childbirth. Trade name is Demerol.

Meprobamate One of the earliest antianxiety tranquilizers. Trade names are Miltown and Equanil.

Merchandise Narcotics.

Mesc Mescaline.

Mesca Marihuana.

Mescal Mescaline.

Mescal Beans Peyote.

Mescal Buttons Peyote.

Mescaline 3,4,5-trimethoxyphenyletylamine, a hallucinogen occurring naturally in heads of peyote cactus. It is also produced synthetically.

Meserole Thick marihuana cigarette; *same as* Panatella.

Message to Garcia Letter that has been written on paper soaked in a narcotics solution and sent to someone in jail.

Metabolism Chemical conversion by enzymes of a drug to other compounds that can be more readily eliminated from the body.

Metabolites Chemical compounds that result from the metabolism of administered drugs.

Meter To feign withdrawal in hopes of convincing a physician to administer or prescribe narcotics.

Meth 1. Methamphetamine hydrochloride. 2. Methadone hydrochloride.

Meth Freak Frequent user of methamphetamine whose life-style revolves around use of the drug.

Meth Head Frequent user of methamphetamine.

Meth Monster *Same as* Meth Head.

Methadone hydrochloride Synthetic narcotic less potent than heroin or morphine that is used in maintenance or detoxification programs for individuals dependent on these drugs. Comes in form of white crystals that are water soluble, or tablets. Trade name is Dolophine.

Methadone maintenance Substitution of methadone for heroin in an effort to decrease dependence on narcotics by permitting user eventually to become drug free. Initiated in 1964.

Methamphetamine hydrochloride The most popular of the amphetamines taken by chronic amphetamine users. Often taken intravenously. Comes in the form of white, orange, and yellow tablets and ampules. Trade names are Methedrine and Desoxyn.

Methapyriline Antihistamine used to adulterate heroin.

Methaqualone Nonbarbiturate sedative/hypnotic first synthesized in 1951. Comes in form of yellow, light orange, and white tablets. Trade names are Mandrax, Quaalude, Sopor, and Somnafac.

Methedrine Methamphetamine hydrochloride.

Methylmorphine Chemical name for codeine.

Methylphenidate hydrochloride Drug mainly used to treat hyperactivity in children. Trade name is Ritalin.

Mex, Mexican Marihuana.

Mexican Brown, Green, Red High-potency marihuana from Mexico.

Mexican Horse Brown heroin from Mexico.

Mexican Mud Brown heroin from Mexico.

Mexican Reds Red Seconal pills imported from Mexico.

Mezz Marihuana cigarette (1930s–1940s). From Milton "Mezz" Mezzrow, jazz clarinetist. Mezzrow sold high-potency marihuana on the streets of Harlem. He was arrested in 1940 for possession and served seventeen months in prison.

Mezz Roll Fat marihuana cigarette (1930s–1940s).

Mezzaine Lover Marihuana user.

Mezzony, Mizzony 1. Money for purchase of marihuana or other drugs. 2. Meeting between buyer and seller of drugs (1930s–1940s).

Mick To give someone a Mickey Finn.

Mickey Small bottle of wine.

Mickey Finn A drink, usually alcohol, to which chloral hydrate has been added.

Mickey Flynn *Same as* Mickey Finn.

Mickey Mouse Habit Irregular use of small amount of drugs.

Microdots LSD.

Microgram One-millionth of a gram.

Middling Acting as a middleman between dealer and buyer.

Midnight Lab Illegal-drug-producing laboratory.

Midnight Oil Opium.

Midnight Oil, Burning the Smoking opium.

Midnight Oil Burner Opium user.

Mig Marihuana.

Miggies Marihuana.

Miggles Marihuana cigarettes.

Mighty Joe Young Barbiturates.

Mighty Mezz Potent marihuana cigarette.

Mighty Quinn LSD.

Mike 1. Any narcotic. 2. Microgram.

Milk Sugar Lactose, a substance used to adulterate heroin or other drugs.

Milligram One-thousandth of a gram.

Milliliter One-thousandth of a liter.

Mind Blower 1. Drug that produces profound sensory distortions. 2. Hallucinogen.

Mind Detergent LSD.

Mind Fuck To give someone a drug, usually a hallucinogen, for the enjoyment of those watching his reaction.

Mind Reader *See* Scopolamine.

Ming Marihuana cigarette made of roaches.

Minibennies Amphetamines.

Minor Tranquilizer Antianxiety tranquilizer.

Mint Leaf PCP.

Mint Weed PCP.

Mired in the Mud Dependent on opium.

Misdemeanor A criminal offense less serious than a felony, the sentence for which may or may not result in a jail term.

Miss Injection intended for a vein but injected instead under skin.

Miss Broad Shoulders Female social worker.

Miss Carrie Drugs hidden in someone's clothes or room to "carry" him to the next need for drugs if his usual place of hiding is discovered.

Miss Emma Morphine.

Miss Emma Jones Morphine.

Miss Morph Morphine.

Miss the Channel To miss injecting the needle into a vein.

Missionary Drug seller who initiates non-drug users into drug use, or agent of drug seller who earns a commission by so doing.

Mist PCP.

Mizzony To meet with a drug seller.

M.J. Marihuana.

MMDA Methoxy-methylene dioxyphenyl isopropylamine, a drug similar in structure and effects to amphetamines.

M.M.'s Marihuana munchies, a craving for food after using marihuana.

M.O. Marihuana.

Modams Marihuana.

Moggles Marihuana cigarettes.

Mohasky Marihuana.

Mohasty Marihuana.

Mojo 1. Cocaine. 2. Any narcotic.

Molasses Crude opium.

Molotov Cocktail Thermos bottle in which the space between the inner and outer layers has been filled with narcotics.

Monkey Narcotics. Reference to carnival monkey act in which monkey held tenaciously onto the back of another animal while it ran around a ring.

Monkey Bait Small free sample of narcotics, given to initiate a newcomer into use.

Monkey Bite Dependence on narcotics.

Monkey Cage Opium den.

Monkey Cocaine Cocaine.

Monkey Doodle Needle marks resulting from intravenous narcotics administration.

Monkey Drill Medicine dropper and pin used to administer narcotics intravenously.

Monkey Dust PCP.

Monkey Heroin Heroin.

Monkey House Opium den.

Monkey in the Closet Secret dependence on narcotics.

Monkey in the Wool Dependence on narcotics.

Monkey Janes Marihuana.

Monkey Jumps Uncoordinated walk of someone under the influence of narcotics.

Monkey Medicine Narcotics.

Monkey Money Money to be used to buy narcotics.

Monkey Morphine Morphine.

Monkey on (One's) Back 1. Dependence on narcotics. 2. In need of narcotics to prevent withdrawal.

Monkey Opium Opium.

Monkey Pump Hypodermic syringe for administering narcotics.

Monkey Scratch Self-inflicted scratch associated with narcotics withdrawal.

Monkey Talk Incomprehensible speech due to the influence of narcotics.

Monkey Wagon Dependence on narcotics.

Monkey Wagon, Jump on the To take narcotics.

Monkey with a Long Tail Prescription calling for a large amount of narcotics.

Monkey with a Short Tail Prescription calling for a small amount of narcotics.

Monkey with Minnows To use drugs that do not produce dependence.

Monroe in a Cadillac Mixture of morphine and cocaine.

Moocah 1. Marihuana. 2. Morphine.

Mooch Narcotics.

Mooster Marihuana.

Mootah Marihuana.

Mooter Marihuana.

Mootie Marihuana.

Mooto Marihuana.

Mor a Grifa Marihuana.

More PCP.

Morfiend Morphine user. From *morphine* and *fiend*.

Morning Glory First administration of narcotics of the day.

Morning-glory seeds Seeds from blue-and-white species of the garden plant morning glory. Seeds contain lysergic acid amide, a hallucinogen, which is related to LSD.

Morph Morphine.

Morphie Morphine.

Morphina Morphine.

Morphine Principal psychoactive constituent of opium. Isolated in 1803. Named after Morpheus, Greek god of dreams. First used extensively during American Civil War, resulting in dependence called the Army Disease.

Morphinomania Craving for morphine.

Morpho Morphine.

Morphy Morphine.

Morshtop Morphine.

Moscop Combination of morphine and scopolamine.

Mosquito Cocaine.

Mother 1. Marihuana. 2. One's drug supplier.

Mother Dear Methamphetamine.

Mother Nature Marihuana.

Mother Nature's Own Tobacco Marihuana.

Moto Marihuana.

Motta Marihuana.

Motter Marihuana.

Mount Someone dependent on narcotics.

Mount Shasta, To Be from To be dependent on drugs.

Mouth Habit Drug dependence that is satisfied by swallowing rather than injecting.

Mouse Informer.

Mr. Broad Shoulders Male social worker.

Mr. Fish Narcotics user who voluntarily commits himself to a treatment center.

Mr. Morpheus Morphine.

Mr. Twenty-six Hypodermic needle. From the gauge of the needle.

Mr. Warner Marihuana smoker.

M.S. Morphine.

Mu Marihuana.

M.U. Marihuana smoker.

Mud 1. Crude opium. 2. Crude marihuana. 3. Hashish. 4. Cocaine paste used in medicine.

Mud, Mired in the Dependent on opium.

Muggles Marihuana cigarettes.

Muggle Head Marihuana smoker.

Muggled Up Under the influence of marihuana.

Mule 1. Drug smuggler hired for money to carry drugs. Not in business for oneself. 2. Marihuana mixed with whiskey.

Munchies Acute hunger sensation experienced after smoking marihuana.

Munsh Opium.

Murder Weed Marihuana.

Muscle To inject intramuscularly.

Muscle relaxer Tranquilizer. Term indicates the initial reason for which these drugs were introduced.

Mushroom Psilocybin.

Musta Marihuana.

Muta Marihuana.

Mutha Marihuana.

Muzzle Heroin.

N

NA *See* Narcotics Anonymous.

Nabilone Synthetic drug with many of the same effects as tetrahydrocannabinol.

Nabs Police.

NACC *See* Narcotic Addiction Control Commission.

Nail 1. Needle or pin used to inject narcotics intravenously. 2. Marihuana cigarette.

Nailed Arrested.

Nailers Police officers.

Nalline Trade name for nalorphine, a narcotic antagonist.

Nalline test Procedure used to determine opiate dependence. Principal of the test is based on Nalline causing the pupils of the eye to increase in size in individuals dependent on narcotics. Usual effect of narcotics is to cause constriction of the pupil. In nondependent individual, Nalline has no effect. In dependent individual, Nalline antagonizes narcotic effect thereby causing dilation of pupils.

Nalorphine Semisynthetic derivative of morphine. Trade name is Nalline. Acts as a narcotic antagonist.

Naloxone challenge *Same as* Nalline test except that naloxone is used.

Naloxone hydrochloride Narcotic antagonist. One of the most common drugs used in cases of narcotics overdose. Primarily used to reverse respiratory depression associated with overdosing. Does not produce tolerance or dependence when taken alone. Produces abrupt withdrawal reactions in those dependent on narcotics. Trade name is Narcan.

Naltrexone Narcotic antagonist with no dependence-producing properties and no euphoria-producing effects.

Nanogram One-billionth of a gram.

NARA *See* Narcotic Addiction Rehabilitation Act.

Narc, Narco, Nark 1. Federal narcotics officer. 2. Undercover agent who associates with drug users to gather evidence, which later will be used against them. 2. Hospital for treatment of narcotic dependence in Lexington, Kentucky.

Narcan Naloxone.

Narco *See* Narc, Narco, Nark.

Narcoland World of the narcotics user.

Narco Rap Prison sentence for violation of narcotics laws.

Narcomania Craving for narcotics.

Narconon Program to reduce drug abuse. Program does not involve drug treatment or psychotherapy. Instead, it helps individual to identify his reasons for drug use and tries to offer other ways of coping with whatever problems caused drug use.

Narcopper Narcotics officer.

Narcosis Sleep; stupor; lack of responsiveness.

Narcotic Any drug that produces narcosis, i.e., depression of the central nervous system. From the Greek *narkotikos*, "stupefying." Pharmacologically, it is generally used as a synonym for opiate drugs.

    Around the turn of the century, *narcotic* came to be used as a synonym for illegal drugs, primarily the opiates. This was later expanded to include cocaine, marihuana, mescaline, and chloral hydrate. The term has also been used as a synonym for drugs that cause dependence and are associated with criminal activity.

Narcotic Addiction Rehabilitation Act of 1966 Federal law established in 1966 which provided for commitment of drug dependent volunteers and eligible offenders for short-term, in-patient treatment or long-term confinement and treatment.

Narcotic Addiction Control Commission New York State agency established in 1966 to oversee the New York Addict Commitment Program. Program allowed for nonpunitive treatment of narcotics users. Agency changed its name in 1973 to the Office of Drug Abuse Services. In 1978 it became the Division of Substance Abuse Services.

Narcotic analgesic *Same as* Narcotic.

Narcotic antagonist Substance that can block the physiological and psychological effects of opiate narcotics, for example, naloxone, nalorphine, naltrexone, cyclazocine. Substances can also precipitate acute withdrawal syndromes in narcotics users. Such precipitation as in the Nalline test, is used to identify dependent individuals for legal or medical purposes.

Narcotic Bulls *Same as* Narc, Narco, Nark.

Narcotic Drug Control Act of 1956 Federal law specifically outlawing heroin and marihuana and establishing mandatory minimum penalties for conviction of offenses. Law also provided death penalty if recommended by jury. Law was replaced in 1970 by the Drug Abuse Act.

Narcotic Limitation Convention of 1931 League of Nations agreement to limit manufacture and distribution of narcotic drugs by each country.

Narcotics Anonymous Self-help group patterned on Alcoholics Anonymous. Formed in 1953.

Narcotics Treatment Administration (NTA) Treatment program for heroin users. Established in 1969 in Washington, D.C. Program involves methadone maintenance, counseling by ex-addicts, outpatient programs, voluntary self-referrals, probation, and parole. Users are referred by D.C. courts and Department of Corrections.

Narcotics Ziph Argot of narcotics users and sellers in which "iz" is inserted into words.

Narcotism Dependence on narcotics.

Nark *See* Narc, Narco, Nark.

Nasal Irrigator Drug paraphernalia used to reduce nasal membrane damage from sniffing cocaine and to enhance sensation of future sniffings.

Natch Trip Intoxication produced from naturally occurring and legal substances, for example, nutmeg, peyote, mushrooms, morning-glory seeds.

National Commission on Marihuana and Drug Abuse Commission appointed in 1971 by President Nixon to evaluate marihuana use in the United States. Proposed decriminalization of marihuana. *See* Shafer Commission.

National Committee on the Treatment of Intractable Pain Nonprofit organization promoting research on pain. Advocates use of heroin to treat pain in some circumstances.

National Drug Abuse Treatment Utilization Survey (NDATUS) Federal survey conducted by NIDA of all drug abuse treatment centers to determine extent of drug abuse in the United States.

National Federation of Parents for Drug Free Youth (NFP) National organization of self-help parent groups formed to help local parent groups discourage illicit drug use among children.

National Formulary Book containing descriptions and chemical formulas of drugs.

National Institute of Mental Health (NIMH) U.S. agency responsible for promoting mental health, prevention and treatment of mental illness, and rehabilitation of the mentally ill.

National Institute on Alcohol Abuse and Alcoholism (NIAAA) U.S. agency responsible for prevention, control, and treatment of alcohol abuse and rehabilitation of alcohol abusers.

National Institute on Drug Abuse (NIDA) U.S. agency responsible for providing means for prevention, control, and treatment of drug abuse. Created in 1973.

National Organization for the Reform of Marihuana Laws (NORML) Washington, D.C., based national lobbying group advocating more lenient marihuana laws at federal and state levels.

National Survey on Drug Abuse Ongoing survey of drug abuse in the United States.

Native American Church Religion followed by American Indians that combines Christianity, native religion, and ritual use of peyote.

Nebbies Nembutal, a barbiturate.

Needle 1. Paraphernalia for intravenous narcotics injection including needle and syringe. 2. Heroin.

Needle Fiend, Needle Freak 1. Narcotics user who injects drug intravenously. 2. Drug user who gets pleasure merely from injecting himself by means of a needle.

Needle Habit Narcotics dependency satisfied by narcotics injection.

Needle Happy Fascination with intravenous injection more than with drug effects per se.

Needle Man Narcotics user who injects drug intravenously.

Needle Park Area of New York City around upper Broadway and Sherman Square that was formerly a gathering place for narcotics users.

Needle Pusher *Same as* Needle Fiend, Freak.

Needle Sharing Sharing the same needle and syringe for injecting narcotics.

Needle Shy Anxious about injecting drugs by needle.

Needle Trouble Difficulty in injecting drugs because of clogged, bent, broken, or dull needle.

Needle Yen Craving for intravenous narcotic injection.

Needled 1. Persuaded to smoke opium. 2. Beginner at injecting drugs.

Nembies Nembutal, a barbiturate.

Nembutal Trade name for pentobarbital sodium, a short-acting barbiturate. Comes in the form of yellow capsule for 30- and 100-milligram doses, and yellow-and-white capsule for 50-milligram dose.

Nemish Nembutal.

Nepalese Hash Potent hashish from Nepal.

Nepalese Temple Balls Balls of hashish used in Hindu religious ceremonies. Now imported for profane use.

Nepalese Temple Hash *Same as* Nepalese Temple Balls.

Nepenthe Drug mentioned by poet Homer in the *Odyssey* (4:219–32); literally "against sorrow." Homer did not specifically identify the drug; various authors have considered it to be opium or marihuana.

Neuroleptic Antipsychotic tranquilizer.

Neurosine Drug preparation containing marihuana. Sold during the 1930s.

Neurotransmitter Chemical messenger between nerves. Various drugs produce their effects by mimicking the actions of these chemicals.

New Magic PCP.

New York White *See* Manhattan Silver.

Nialamide Antidepressant. Trade name is Niamid.

Nickel 1. Five-year jail sentence. 2. About three "matchheads" of PCP.

Nickel Bag Five-dollar packet of heroin or marihuana.

Nicotine Principal active ingredient in tobacco. Considered responsible for the smoking habit.

NIDA *See* National Institute on Drug Abuse.

Niebla PCP.

Nimbies Nembutal, a barbiturate.

Nimby Nembutal, a barbiturate.

Nitric acid test Field test for suspected narcotics using nitric acid.

Nitrous Nitrous oxide.

Nitrous oxide Short-acting colorless gaseous anesthetic. Also called laughing gas. Used as an aerosol propellant. Can produce exhilaration and euphoria initially with light use. Heavier use can produce uncoordination and analgesia.

Nixon Low-potency narcotics.

No Name Cigarette Marihuana cigarette.

Nob of Salt Narcotics concealed in top of saltshaker by drug seller who works in a restaurant and passes drugs to buyer in this way.

Noble Princess of the Waters Psilocybin.

Noble Weed Marihuana.

Nocks Narcotics.

Nockskeller Place where narcotics are purchased.

Noctec Trade name for chloral hydrate.

Nod, on the *Same as* Nodding.

Nodding Semistuporous state associated with drug use, characterized by bobbing or bowed head, drooping eyelids, and dozing.

Noise Heroin.

Nonhustling Dope Fiend Drug user who supports his habit by begging rather than criminal activity.

Nonmedical drug use Nontherapeutic use of drugs.

NORML *See* National Organization for the Reform of Marihuana Laws.

Nose 1. Cocaine. 2. Heroin.

Nose Burner Butt of marihuana cigarette.

Nose Candy Cocaine.

Nose Habit Practice of sniffing drugs.

Nose Powder Cocaine.

Nose Stuff Cocaine.

Nose Warmer *Same as* Nose Burner.

Nowhere Without any money or drugs.

Nuggets Amphetamines.

Numbed Out Very intoxicated by PCP, to the point of experiencing bodily anesthesia.

Number Marihuana cigarette.

Number Eight Heroin. From *h*, the eighth letter of the alphabet.

Number Thirteen Morphine. From *m*, the thirteenth letter of the alphabet.

Number Three Cocaine. From *c*, the third letter of the alphabet.

Number Two Sale Second conviction for sale of narcotics.

Nut, Nutmeg East Indian evergreen seeds. Causes mild, brief euphoria, lightheadedness, floating feelings, and CNS excitation. High doses cause fast heartbeat, thirst, nervousness, and sometimes panic. Used by prisoners and sailors. Active ingredient is myristicin.

O

O 1. Ounce of drugs. 2. Opium.

Oaxacan Potent marihuana from the Mexican state of Oaxaca.

Occupational User Individual who feels that he/she cannot perform job without drugs.

O.D. Overdose. Administration of a quantity of drug greater than that normally used. Generally used in reference to narcotic dose that results in death. Sometimes used to indicate drug dose resulting in unpleasant reaction.

ODALE *See* Office of Drug Abuse Law Enforcement.

Odyssey House Therapeutic program for drug addicts. Strives for changes in behavior and attitudes about drugs. Has professional and ex–drug-user staff and has in-residence stage followed by re-entry. Funded by federal and state governments and private donations.

Off Intoxicated by a drug.

Off Brand Cigarette Marihuana cigarette.

Office of Drug Abuse Law Enforcement (ODALE) Established in 1972, the agency was responsible for development and enforcement of federal drug abuse laws. It was abolished in 1973.

Ogoy Heroin.

Ohio Bag Bag containing 100 grams of marihuana—the quantity that qualifies as the maximum amount allowed for a simple possession fine under Ohio's decriminalization law.

Oil 1. Hashish oil. 2. Heroin.

Oil Burner Narcotics user who needs a large amount of drug to satisfy his dependency.

Oil Burning Habit Dependence on narcotics.

Oiler Hashish oil user.

O.J. Opium joint; marihuana dipped in liquid opium. Popular in Vietnam.

Old Lady White Narcotics.

Old Lady's Place Place where narcotics are used.

Old Madge Cocaine.

Old Steve 1. Heroin. 2. Morphine. 3. Cocaine.

Olive Cotton used to filter dissolved narcotics.

On Under the influence of a drug.

On the Beam Intoxicated by marihuana.

On the Gow Dependent on narcotics.

On the Mojo Dependent on narcotics.

On the Natch Abrupt and unsupervised narcotics withdrawal.

On the Needle Dependent on narcotics involving intravenous administration.

On the Nod *Same as* Nodding.

On the Pipe Dependent on opium.

On the Point Staring into space as a result of taking methamphetamines.

On the Stuff 1. Using heroin. 2. Dependent on a drug.

On the Wrong End of the Bamboo Opium smoker.

On Top of It In control.

One, the *Same as* Hash Oil. Succeeded in 1971 by Son of One.

One and One Using both nostrils to inhale a drug.

One-hit Grass DMT.

One-toke Weed Marihuana so potent that only a few inhalations produce intoxication.

Op, Ope Opium.

Operation Intercept U.S. attempt to shut off the flow of marihuana from Mexico in 1969. The project was abandoned twenty days after initiation, after protests from the Mexican government and American citizens who were subjected to searches and long traffic jams at border.

Operator Drug seller.

Opiated Hash Hashish to which opium has been added.

Opiates Compounds including opium, the opium alkaloids (morphine and codeine), and those derived from them, such as heroin.

Opioids Synthetic derivatives of morphine and codeine such as meperidine and methadone.

Opium The milky residue obtained from cut, unripe seed pods of the opium poppy, *Papaver somniferum*. Contains morphine and codeine.

Opium Joint Place where opium is smoked.

Opium Kippers Opium smokers lying on bunks in an opium den.

Opium Protocol of 1953 United Nations agreement to limit opium production and export. Production was limited to Bulgaria, Greece, India, Iran, Turkey, Russia, and Yugoslavia. Only licensed farmers were allowed to cultivate opium, and production was solely to be used for medical and scientific needs.

Opiumery Place where opium is smoked.

Optimil Methaqualone.

Orange Dexedrine. Term based on color of tablet.

Orange Crystal PCP.

Orange Cubes LSD.

Orange Micro LSD.

Orange Mushroom LSD.

Orange Owsley LSD.

Orange Sunshine LSD.

Orange Wedges LSD.

Oranges Amphetamines.

Oregano Herb resembling marihuana. Used to dilute marihuana or to deceive naive buyers.

Oregon Decriminalization Bill First (1973) state law decriminalizing marihuana from a felony to a $100 civil misdemeanor.

Oriental Dreamer Opium smoker.

Ossified Very intoxicated by a drug.

OTC Drugs *See* Over-the-counter Drugs.

Ounce Man Large-scale narcotics distributor. *Same as* Connection.

Out No longer intoxicated by marihuana.

Out of It 1. No longer using drugs. 2. Very intoxicated by a drug.

Out of Sight Excellent; superior; first-rate.

Outer 1. LSD. 2. Mescaline.

Outfit Paraphernalia for intravenous injection. *Same as* Artillery.

Over the Hump 1. Beyond the most difficult part of withdrawal from narcotics. 2. Beyond the most euphoric period associated with drug use.

Over the Top No longer dependent on narcotics.

Overamped Taken an overdose of a stimulant.

Overcharged Under the influence of a larger-than-usual dose of narcotics.

Overdose *See* O.D.

Overdosed Totally overcome by PCP to the point of loss of consciousness.

Overjolt *Same as* O.D.

Over-the-counter Drugs Drugs that can be purchased without a prescription.

Owsley LSD. From August Stanley Owsley III, a chemist who produced the drug illegally.

Owsley's Acid LSD.

Owsley's Blue Dot LSD.

Oxazepam Antianxiety tranquilizer. Trade name is Serax. A member of the Valium group of drugs.

Oxycodone hydrochloride Semisynthetic derivative of codeine. Trade names are Percodan, Percocet–5, and Tylox.

OZ Brand name for amyl nitrite.

O.Z. Ounce of drug.

Ozone PCP.

Ozone, in the Intoxicated by marihuana.

Ozoned Very intoxicated by PCP. Effects include incoherence and immobility.

P

P 1. PCP. 2. Peyote.

Pack Heroin.

Pack (of Rockets, of Rocks) Package of marihuana cigarettes.

Pack (One's) Keyster To conceal drugs in the rectum, usually inside a condom.

Packed Up Intoxicated by a drug.

Pad 1. Place where drugs are used. 2. Room, apartment, sleeping quarters.

Paid Off in Gold Arrested by an undercover federal narcotics agent after selling him drugs. After paying for and receiving drugs, agent produces his badge.

Pakistani Hash Potent hashish from Pakistan.

Pan Juice Crude opium.

Pan Yen Opium.

Panama Canal Zone Military Inquiry First (1916–1929) official U.S. inquiry into the effects of marihuana. The investigation centered on marihuana usage by American soldiers serving in the Panama Canal Zone. The inquiry contained the first officially conducted laboratory experiments on the effects of marihuana on human subjects.

Panama Gold Potent marihuana from Panama, gold in color.

Panama Red Potent marihuana from Panama, red in color.

Panatella 1. Thickly rolled marihuana cigarette. Originally an expensive cigar. 2. Potent marihuana sold for twenty-five cents per cigarette in 1940s.

Pangonadalot Heroin.

Panic 1. Scarcity of narcotics. 2. In need of narcotics.

Panic Man 1. Narcotics seller. 2. Narcotics user in need of drugs.

Panic reaction Adverse reaction to psychoactive drugs characterized by fear, anxiety, and sometimes inability to move.

Papaver somniferum Botanical name for poppy plant from which
opium and its derivatives are obtained.

Papaverine Naturally occurring constituent of opium that causes
depression of the heartbeat and smooth muscle activity. Does not
produce analgesia or affect the brain as do morphine and codeine,
two other constituents of opium.

Paper 1. Small amount of narcotics. 2. Paper soaked in a solution of
narcotics and then dried. Used to smuggle narcotics into prison.
3. Prescription. 4. LSD solution on paper.

Paper Acid LSD solution on paper.

Papers Cigarette papers used to make marihuana cigarettes.

Parackie Paraldehyde.

Paradise Cocaine.

Paral Paraldehyde.

Paraldehyde Nonbarbiturate sedative/hypnotic synthesized in 1829.
Introduced into medicine in 1882. Colorless, bitter liquid. Previ-
ously used to treat delirium tremens.

Paraldy Paraldehyde.

Paranoia Condition characterized by extreme suspiciousness, and fear
of being arrested.

Paraphernalia Equipment and material used to administer or store
illegal drugs or to make them more potent.

Paraquat Herbicide used to eradicate marihuana fields.

Paregoric Tincture containing about 4 percent opium. Introduced
during the early eighteenth century. Primarily used to control
diarrhea. Resorted to by narcotics users when heroin or morphine
are unavailable.

Parenteral Drug administration by hypodermic injection.

Parest Methaqualone.

Park Land Number Twos Marihuana from Cambodia; term used
by Americans in Vietnam.

Parsley PCP.

Party 1. Gathering of two or more people at which drugs are taken.
2. To socialize and use drugs.

Partying Any planned gathering at which drugs are used.

Passed Out Unconscious as a result of alcohol intoxication or drug use.

Passed Out of the Picture *Same as* Passed Out.

Paste Coca paste.

Pasted Dependent on narcotics.

Pasty Face Narcotics user. Term derived from pale complexion of narcotics user.

Patent Medicine Drug protected by patent from being copied as to name, composition, or method of manufacture.

Pato de gayina Literally "feet of chicken." Form of sinsemilla. So called because of shape of pod.

Pattern of drug use Amount of drug use and situations it is used in, for example, experimental, recreational, compulsive, circumstantial, social.

PAZ PCP.

PCE Analog of PCP. Chemical name is N-ethyl-1-phenylcyclohexylamine hydrochloride.

PCP Phencyclidine. Trade name is Sernyl. Chemical name is 1-(1-phencyclohexyl) piperidine hydrochloride. Sold in the form of a white crystal or powder that can be injected, smoked, or mixed with other drugs, in the form of a tablet or capsule, or dissolved in liquid. Sometimes placed on parsley, oregano, tobacco, mint, or marihuana, and smoked. Administered orally, by smoking in conjunction with marihuana, by snorting, rectally, or vaginally. Also taken in eye drops. Produces both stimulant and depressant effects as well as hallucinogenic effects.

  Became popular in 1967 although synthesized as early as 1926. Drug trials conducted under the name Sernyl by pharmaceutical firm of Parke, Davis and Company. Initially of interest because it produced deep anesthesia without causing loss of consciousness in animals. Manufacture was discontinued due to adverse side effects in humans. Introduced as a "street drug" around 1967. Became popular around 1973. Easily manufactured by underground chemists. Effects associated with lower doses ("buzzed" state) are mild euphoria and stimulation. Higher dose produces slurred speech, uncoordination, and speeding up of thought processes ("wasted" state). Higher dose produces immobility but not loss of consciousness ("ozoned" state). Next higher state produces loss of consciousness, possible convulsions, coma, and death ("overdosed" state).

PCPA PCP.

PCPY Analog of PCP. Chemical name is 1-(1-phenylcyclohexyl) pyr-
rolidine hydrochloride.

Pea Ce Pill PCP.

Peace 1. PCP. 2. LSD. 3. STP.

Peace Tablets LSD.

Peaceweed PCP.

Peaches Benzedrine tablets. From the color.

Peanut Butter PCP added to peanut butter.

Peanuts Barbiturates.

Pearl Amyl nitrite ampule.

Pearly Gates 1. LSD. 2. Morning-glory seeds.

Pearly Whites Morning-glory seeds.

Pekoe High-potency opium.

Pellets LSD.

Pellicle High-potency opium.

Pemoline Stimulant. White, tasteless, odorless powder or tablet.

Pen Shot *Abbreviation for* Penitentiary Shot.

Pen Yen Opium.

Penitentiary Shot *Same as* Pin Shot.

Pentazocine hydrochloride Synthetic narcotic drug produced in
early 1960s. Trade name is Talwin. Initially thought to be non–
dependence-producing analgesic equal to morphine. Subse-
quently found to produce dependence. Also has narcotic antago-
nism properties.

Pentobarbital sodium Short-acting barbiturate. Trade name is
Nembutal.

Pentothal sodium Short-acting barbiturate. Often used in combination with other drugs. In small amounts causes suggestibility.
Used by police as "truth serum."

Pep Pills Amphetamines.

Pep-em-ups Amphetamines.

Pepsi-Cola Habit Use of only a small amount of narcotics.

Per Prescription.

Percobarb Combination of Percodan and a barbiturate.

Percodan Codeine derivative. Used medicinally for pain relief. Comes
in form of yellow or light purple pills.

Percs Percodan.

Perico Cocaine.

Period Hitter Irregular narcotics user.

Perks Percodan.

Persian Dust Heroin.

Personal Hash Hashish sold only to other dealers for personal use; very potent.

Pete *Same as* Sneaky Pete.

Peter 1. Narcotics. 2. Chloral hydrate.

Peter Pan PCP.

Pethidine *See* Meperidine hydrochloride.

Peyote 1. Peyote, cactus plant (*Lophophora williamsii*) whose main psychoactive ingredient is mescaline. 2. PCP.

Peyote Button Tip of the peyote cactus. Contains the hallucinogen mescaline.

Peyotyl Peyote.

P.G. Paregoric.

Phantastica Drugs producing altered perceptions in which the user is aware of what he is experiencing and can remember what has been experienced, for example, peyote, LSD.

Pharmacogenic Orgasm Term coined in 1926 by S. Rado to refer to pleasurable feeling in the stomach experienced by heroin users following intravenous heroin injection.

Pharmacokinetics Study of the absorption, distribution, metabolism, and elimination of drugs from the body.

Pharmacology Study of the effects of drugs.

Phencyclidine *See* PCP.

Phenmetrazine hydrochloride Stimulant. Trade name is Preludin.

Phennies Phenobarbital.

Pheno Phenobarbital.

Phenobarbital Long-acting barbiturate. Trade name is Luminal.

Phoenix House Rehabilitation center for heroin users.

Phenotype Visible characteristics of genetic inheritance.

Phenotypic ratio Method of classifying different variants of marihuana according to the ratio of three main cannabinoids—delta-9-tetrahydrocannabinol, cannabinol, and cannabidiol.

Phonies Fake drugs containing inert or poisonous material.

PHP Phenylcyclohexylpyrrolidine, an analog of PCP.

Physical dependence *See* Dependence.

Physician's Desk Reference Comprehensive book about drugs and their effects.

Pick Up 1. To smoke marihuana. 2. To take narcotics.

Pick Up Smoking Sharing a marihuana cigarette.

Picking the Poppies Dependent on opium.

Piddle Hospital where narcotics users are treated.

Piece 1. Ounce of a drug. 2. Cocaine. 3. Morphine. 4. Heroin.

Pig 1. Police officer. 2. Container for opium.

Pig Killer PCP.

Pig Outfit Clandestine laboratory manufacturing PCP.

Pig Rap Discussion among drug users about police harassment.

Pig Tranquilizer PCP.

Pigfoot Marihuana.

Piggie Amount of opium prepared for smoking.

Piki Opium.

Pill 1. Pellet of opium. After opium has been "cooked," it takes the shape of a round pill. 2. Barbiturate.

Pill Addict Chronic barbiturate user.

Pill Baby Female chronic barbiturate user.

Pill Cooker 1. Opium user. 2. Person who prepares opium for smoking.

Pill Freak Chronic pill user whose life-style revolves around using pills, in any amount at any time.

Pill Head Chronic user of barbiturates or amphetamines.

Pill Popper Someone who swallows numerous drugs.

Pillman Someone who combines barbiturates with alcohol.

Pillow 1. Opium. 2. Methaqualone.

Pills Barbiturates.

Pimp Dust Cocaine.

Pin Thin marihuana cigarette.

Pin Gun Paraphernalia for intravenous injection consisting of an eyedropper and a pin.

Pin Head Narcotics user who uses an eyedropper and pin instead of a hypodermic syringe and needle.

Pin Shot Intravenous narcotics injection using an eyedropper and a pin. The pin is used to open the vein and the dropper is then applied to the wound.

Pinch Quantity of marihuana. About enough to make two cigarettes.

Ping Lang Betel nuts.

Ping in the Wing Injection into the arm.

Pinhead Thin marihuana cigarette.

Pink Darvon.

Pink Ladies Seconal, a barbiturate.

Pink Owsley LSD.

Pink Swirl LSD.

Pink Wedge LSD.

Pinks Seconal, a barbiturate. From the color of the capsule.

Pinned Constricted pupils of the eyes resulting from heroin use.

Pinner *Same as* Pin.

Pipe Large vein.

Pipe, Riding the Smoking opium.

Pipe Dream Dream produced by opium.

Pipe Factory Opium den.

Pipe Fiend Chronic opium smoker.

Pipe Hitter *Same as* Pipe Fiend.

Piperidine Precursor of PCP.

Pipradol benzilate A hallucinogen.

Pipy Opium smoker.

Pit Primary vein going to the heart.

Pital *Same as* Piddle.

Pitch To sell narcotics.

Pixies Amphetamines.

Placebo Inert material.

Plant 1. To place drugs among someone's property so that they will later be found and used as evidence of possession. 2. Informant. 3. Place where narcotics paraphernalia are hidden.

Plants Mescaline.

Play Around To use drugs irregularly.

Play the Clown To pretend to undergo narcotics withdrawal to enlist sympathy from a physician who may then administer narcotics.

Played Completely smoked.

Player Drug user.

Playing the Mouth Organ Inhaling smoke from heated heroin no. 3 through a matchbox cover. Practice used mainly in Hong Kong, where heroin is more potent than that used in United States. Comparable effects can therefore be experienced by inhalation that would require injection of more dilute material (about 5 percent pure heroin) available in United States.

Pleasure Smoker Irregular opium user.

Pleiku Pink Marihuana. Term used by American soldiers in Vietnam.

P.O. Paregoric.

Poco Small amount of narcotics.

Pod Marihuana.

Pogo Pogo Cocaine.

Point Needle.

Point Shot *See* Pin Shot.

Poison 1. Heroin. 2. Cocaine. 3. Informer.

Poison Act *See* Harrison Narcotics Act.

Poke Inhalation of marihuana or opium smoke.

Poking Smoking marihuana or opium.

Policeman Antabuse.

Polluted Under the influence of narcotics.

Polvo PCP.

Polvo de Angel PCP.

Polydrug use Use of a number of different drugs in combination or sequentially.

Pop 1. Injection of narcotics. 2. To swallow a drug.

Pop Stick Homemade opium pipe.

Popo Ore Potent marihuana from Mexico.

Popped Arrested.

Popper Amyl nitrite ampule.

Poppied Under the influence of opium.

Poppies, Picking the Dependent on opium.

Poppy Opium.

Poppy Alley Area of city where opium is used or sold.

Poppy Grove Place where opium is smoked.

Poppy Head Chronic user of opium.

Poppy Rain Opium.

Poppy Train Opium.

Popsie Amyl nitrite ampule.

Possession Possession of a restricted drug with the intent to sell it.

Pot Marihuana.

Pot Head Frequent marihuana smoker.

Pot Likker, Liquor Tea brewed with marihuana.

Pot Lush Chronic marihuana smoker.

Pot Out To smoke marihuana.

Pot Party Gathering at which marihuana is smoked.

Potency Strength of action. The smaller the amount of drug needed to produce a particular effect, the greater its potency.

Potentiation Combined effect of two or more drugs such that the combination produces a greater effect than either alone. *See also* Additive effect; *same as* Synergism.

Potted Under the influence of marihuana.

Pound Action Buying a pound of marihuana.

Powder 1. Marihuana; hashish. 2. Heroin. 3. Amphetamine in powdered form. 4. Cocaine.

Powder Diamonds Cocaine.

Powdered 1. Under the influence of cocaine. 2. Intoxicated by alcohol.

Powdered Bread Money that has been secretly marked and is used by police to buy drugs.

Powdered Joy Narcotics.

Power Hit Inhaling smoke from a marihuana cigarette and then blowing it into another smoker's mouth as he inhales.

Pox Opium pill.

P.R. Panama Red. Potent marihuana from Panama, red in color.

Prescription Written request by a physician for dispensing a drug, along with instructions for its use.

Prescription Reds Any drug in a red capsule.

President Johnson's Commission on Law Enforcement and

Administration Commission appointed by President Johnson in 1967 to study drug laws. Commission urged distinction between narcotics and marihuana.

President Kennedy's Ad Hoc Panel on Drug Abuse Panel appointed by President Kennedy in 1962 to study the drug abuse problem in the United States.

President's Advisory Commission on Narcotics and Drug Abuse Commission appointed in 1963 by President Kennedy to review drug problem in the United States. The commission recommended that minimum mandatory sentences as prescribed by the Boggs Act be reconsidered; that the Bureau of Narcotics be transferred from the Treasury Department to the Department of Health, Education and Welfare; and that increased money be allocated for research into the effects of marihuana. It also recommended that marihuana be differentiated from narcotics.

Prettyman Commission *Same as* President's Advisory Commission on Narcotics and Drug Abuse.

Prick Hypodermic needle.

Prime the Pump To buy narcotics.

Primed to the Ears Having taken a very large amount of narcotics.

Primo First rate; excellent.

Principal active ingredient *See* Active ingredient, principal.

Procaine Local anesthetic used to dilute cocaine.

Proctor and Gamble Paregoric. From the abbreviation P.G.

Prod Narcotics injection.

Prod of Joy *Same as* Prod.

Prodder Narcotics user who injects drug intravenously.

Product IV Combination of LSD and PCP.

Prong Hypodermic needle.

Prop Hypodermic injection.

Proprietary drug Drug protected by patent with regard to trade name, means of manufacture, or composition.

Propxyphene hydrochloride Narcotic analgesic. Trade name is Darvon.

P.S. Opium. From *Papaver somniferum*.

Psilocin Hallucinogen found in *Psilocybe mexicana* mushroom along with psilocybin. Also a metabolite of psilocybin.

Psilocybin Hallucinogen found in mushroom *Psilocybe mexicana*.

Psychedelic Mind-expanding. Term invented by Humphrey Osmond in correspondence with Aldous Huxley in 1956. From Greek *psyche* (soul) and *delos* (visible).

Psychoactive Any drug that acts on the mind.

Psychodysleptic Mind-distorting.

Psychological dependence *See* Dependence.

Psycholytic Mind-loosening.

Psychopharmacology Branch of pharmacology concerned with drugs that affect behavior or subjective experience.

Psychosis Severe mental disturbance in which individual loses touch with reality and may experience hallucinations or delusions.

Psychotraxic Hallucinogenic.

Psychotogenic Producing hallucinations.

Psychotomimetic Substance capable of initiating activity in the brain.

Psychotropic *Same as* Psychoactive.

Puff Opium.

Puff on the Side To smoke opium while lying on one's side.

Puff the Dust To smoke hashish.

Puffing Smoking opium.

Puffy PCP.

Pug Narcotics user trying to abstain.

Pula Seconal.

Pulaski Marihuana smoker.

Pulborn, Pulboron Heroin.

Pull 1. Deep inhalation of smoke from a marihuana cigarette. 2. A drink.

Pump Full of Junk To take a large amount of narcotics.

Punk Low-potency marihuana.

Punta Roja Literally "red point." Potent marihuana from Colombia.

Pure Heroin.

Pure Food and Drug Act (1906) U.S. law that required all patent medicines shipped across state lines to list their ingredients if they contained more than a specified amount of certain drugs.

Pure Love LSD.

Purple Barrels LSD.

Purple Flats LSD.

Purple Haze LSD.

Purple Hearts 1. Amphetamines. 2. Luminal (phenobarbital). From color and shape of tablet.

Purple Microdots LSD.

Purple Passion Combination stimulants and depressants.

Purple Ozoline LSD.

Purring Like a Kitten Feeling euphoric following narcotics use.

Push Shorts To sell a smaller amount of drugs than was paid for.

Pusher Drug seller. Usually used in reference to narcotics, whereas *dealer* is a term used to refer to a marihuana seller. Sometimes also used to refer to a marihuana seller.

Put It in Writing To split a postcard, hide narcotics in the seam, and then reseal the postcard. Method of smuggling drugs into prison.

Put Me Straight Sell me some narcotics.

Put On a Circus To feign withdrawal in hopes of convincing a physician to administer or prescribe narcotics.

Put the Bee On To beg for narcotics.

Puti Methaqualone.

Q

Quaalude Methaqualone. Trade name for drug manufactured by Rorer pharmaceutical company.

Quacks Methaqualone.

Quad Methaqualone.

Quarry Cure Sudden withdrawal from narcotics.

Quarter Bag Quarter-ounce of marihuana.

Quarter Moon Hashish.

Quarter Ounce One-fourth of an ounce of a drug.

Quarter Piece Quarter-ounce of drugs.

Quas Methaqualone.

Quill Matchbook cover on which narcotics are placed and then snorted.

Quinine Drug used to adulterate heroin.

R

Racehorse Charlie 1. Narcotics user. 2. Heroin. 3. Cocaine.

Racked Intoxicated by marihuana.

Raggedy Ann LSD solution on paper.

Ragweed Marihuana.

Rail *Same as* Line.

Railroad Weed Marihuana.

Rainbow Tuinal, a combination of amobarbital and secobarbital powder in a red-and-white capsule.

Rainbow Roll Collection of barbiturate capsules. Term derives from the many colors of the capsules.

Rainy Day Woman Marihuana.

Raise a Welt To make a vein prominent so that drugs can be injected into it.

Raise It To obtain enough money to buy drugs.

Rama Marihuana. Literally "branch" in Spanish.

Rams Delirium tremens.

Rane Cocaine.

Rangoon Marihuana.

Rap 1. To talk. 2. Conversation.

Rare To inhale heroin or cocaine through the mouth.

Raspberry Abscess at site of narcotics injection.

Rastafarians Black Jamaican religious cult that regarded Haile Selassie, whose name was Ras Tafari before he became emperor of Ethiopia, as the living God. The Rastafarians call themselves black Hebrews and Lions of Judah and regard themselves as one of the ten lost tribes of Israel. They take the Biblical verse "Thou shall eat the herb of the field" as a reference to marihuana (*ganja*) and take it in their tea or smoke it as a religious sacrament.

Rat 1. To inform. 2. Informer.

Rat Poison Heroin to which a toxin has been added.

Ration Amount of narcotics used by drug taker in each injection.

Rat-tail Cure Slow withdrawal from narcotics effected by gradually reducing the dose.

R.D.'s *Abbreviation for* Red Devils, Seconal, a barbiturate.

Reach the Pitch To pass beyond the most painful period of narcotics withdrawal.

Reader Prescription for narcotics.

Reader with a Long Tail Prescription for a large amount of narcotics that is being traced by narcotics agents.

Reader with a Short Tail Prescription for a small amount of narcotics that is being traced by narcotics agents.

Reader with a Tail Prescription for narcotics that is being traced by narcotics agents.

Real Hustling Dope Fiend Drug user who supports his habit by criminal activity rather than begging.

Reaper Marihuana.

Receptor Site on cell surface with which some drugs, such as the narcotics, react to initiate activity in the brain.

Recreational drug Drug regarded as benign and controllable; "soft" drug, for example, marihuana, in contrast to "hard" drug, for example, heroin.

Recreational drug use Social or situational use of drugs as opposed to compulsive use.

Red *Abbreviation for* Panama Red.

Red Birds Seconal, a barbiturate.

Red Bullets Seconal, a barbiturate.

Red Chicken Heroin.

Red Cross Morphine. From its use as a painkiller during world wars I and II.

Red Devils *Same as* Red Bullets.

Red Dirt Marihuana Uncultivated, wild marihuana.

Red Dolls Seconal, a barbiturate.

Red Gunyon Powdered marihuana seed pods smoked in a water pipe.

Red Jacket Seconal, a barbiturate.

Red Leb(anese) Potent hashish originating in Lebanon, reddish in color.

Red Lillies Seconal, a barbiturate.

Red Oil Hash oil.

Red Rock Heroin.

Reds Seconal, a barbiturate. From the color of the capsule.

Reds and Blues Tuinal.

Reds and Grays Darvon.

Reducing Pills Amphetamines. So called because they were once prescribed for weight loss.

Reef *Abbreviation for* Reefer.

Reefer Marihuana cigarette. Most common term for marihuana in the 1930s. The term possibly derived from Mexican *grifa*, or *grifo*, which originally meant "someone intoxicated." Owing to the Mexican tendency to elide the *g* at the beginning of a word, *grifa* became *rifa*. When picked up by Americans, *rifa* became *reefa*, and then *reefer*.

Reefer Hound Marihuana smoker.

Reefer Madness 1938 movie about alleged evils of marihuana. Now a cult film.

Reefer Man Marihuana seller.

Reefing Man Marihuana smoker.

Re-entry To come out of a drug treatment experience.

Refreshments Narcotics.

Register To pull back on the syringe, allowing blood to flow into it so that the drug user knows that the needle is in a vein.

Regulation Control rather than prohibition of drug use.

Reindeer Dust Cocaine.

Reserpine Antipsychotic tranquilizer. Isolated from snakeroot (*Rauwolfia serpentina*).

Reverse tolerance Increased sensitivity to a drug as a result of previous usage. Opposite of tolerance.

R.F.D. Junker Narcotics user who approaches country doctors for narcotics.

Rhythms Amphetamines.

Riding the Pipe Smoking opium.

Riding the Poppy Train Dependent on opium.

Riding the Wave Under the influence of narcotics.

Riding the White Horse Drug-induced dreaming.

Riding the Witch's Broom Dependent on heroin.

Rifle Range Ward of hospital where narcotics withdrawal takes place.

Rig Paraphernalia for intravenous injection. *Same as* Artillery.

Right Croaker Physician who sells narcotics or prescriptions for narcotics to users.

Righteous 1. Unadulterated; pure; honest. 2. Good, pleasurable.

Righteous Bush Marihuana.

Righteous Dealer Honest marihuana seller.

Righteous Scoffer Someone who eats ravenously after going through withdrawal.

Rinsings Residue obtained from the cotton used to strain heroin solution.

Rip Off 1. To cheat or steal. 2. A person who cheats or steals.

Rip Offs Fake drugs.

Ripped Physically and psychologically exhausted from extended use of amphetamines.

Rippers Amphetamines.

Ripping and Running *Same as* Taking Care of Business.

Ritalin Mild stimulant with antidepressant properties. Clinically used to treat hyperactivity in children and depression or apathy in adults.

Rizla Brand of marihuana cigarette paper.

Roach Marihuana cigarette butt. So called because the butt has the appearance of a cockroach to some smokers.

Roach Bender Marihuana smoker.

Roach Clip Device used to hold a burning marihuana cigarette butt.

Roach Holder *Same as* Roach Clip.

Roach Pick *Same as* Roach Clip.

Road Dope Amphetamines.

Roast the Beans To prepare opium for smoking.

Robe Robitussin, a cough syrup containing codeine.

Rock 1. Irregularly shaped crystals of cocaine. Less pure than flake. 2. Heroin granules.

Rock Out To fall asleep because of smoking too much marihuana.

Rock Pile Cure Treatment of narcotics dependence by abstinence and hard work.

Rocket Marihuana.

Rocket Fuel 1. Poor-quality PCP. Yellowish, moist, and coarse-looking. 2. Combination of PCP and marihuana.

Roll Package containing a number of pills.

Roll (Up) To make a marihuana cigarette.

Roll a Pill To prepare opium for smoking.

Roll a Stick To make a marihuana cigarette.

Roll in Black Stuff To smoke opium.

Roll the Boy To smoke opium.

Roll the Log To smoke opium.

Roller Vein that moves during injection.

Rolling Buzz Mild intoxication experienced some time after smoking marihuana.

Rolling Machine Device for rolling marihuana cigarettes.

Rolling Paper Extra wide cigarette paper used primarily for making marihuana cigarettes. Currently there are three hundred to four hundred different brands available, ranging in price from ten cents to one dollar a package. Papers may be flavored, for example, strawberry, banana, grape; are made from different kinds of material, for example, wheat, rice; and may be printed, for example, with cartoons.

Rooster Brand Poor-quality opium.

Root Marihuana cigarette.

Root Tonic Opium dissolved in medicinal tonic.

Rope Marihuana. So called because most rope was initially made from hemp, the fibers of the marihuana plant.

Rosa Maria Marihuana.

Rosas Amphetamines.

Rosebud Swollen, painful rectum, as a result of evacuation of hard fecal matter following opium use.

Rosenbloom *Same as* Rosebud.

Roses Benzedrine, an amphetamine.

Rough Stuff Uncleaned marihuana containing seeds and stems.

Round Order of drinks for everyone in a group.

Round the Bend Beyond the most painful part of the process of withdrawal from narcotics.

Rowdy Glue sniffer.

Royal Blues LSD.

Rubber Pill Finger of a rubber glove into which narcotics are put. Glove is then hidden in the rectum.

Run Prolonged period of drug use. Usually used in reference to drugs such as amphetamines.

Runner Delivery man for drug seller.

Running Amok *Same as* Amuck, Amok.

Rush Intense euphoria from drug use. Initially used in reference to effects of narcotics injection.

S

Sack Bag of heroin.

Sacrament LSD.

Sacred Mushroom Psilocybin.

Saddle and Bridle Paraphernalia for smoking opium.

Safety Safety pin used as a makeshift needle for intravenous narcotics injection.

Safety Pin Mechanic Narcotics user who injects drug with a pin and an eyedropper instead of a hypodermic needle and syringe.

Sagebrush Whacker Marihuana smoker.

Salad Combination of drugs.

Salt Heroin.

Salt and Pepper 1. Weak marihuana. 2. Marihuana adulterated with oregano.

Salt Shot Intravenous injection of salt in water, given by friends to a heroin user who has taken an overdose, in the belief that this will revive him.

Sam Federal narcotics officer; from "Uncle Sam."

Sam How Second or third cooking of opium scrapings sold to users who dilute it in water and inject it.

San Lo Poor-quality opium.

San Pedro Cactus Cactus that contains mescaline.

Sand Sugar.

Sandoz LSD. From the name of the company where the drug was first synthesized.

Santa Maria Gold Potent marihuana from Colombia, gold in color.

Santa Maria Red Potent marihuana from Colombia, red in color.

SAODAP *See* Special Action Office for Drug Abuse Prevention.

Sass-fras Weak marihuana cigarette made from marihuana grown in the United States. Term used during the 1940s.

Satan's Apple Mandrake.

Satan's Scent Brand name for amyl nitrite.

Satch Drugs concealed by saturating absorbent material, for example, clothes, with them, so that if arrested, drugs will still be available.

Satch Cotton Cotton used to filter narcotics before injection. Cotton is saved and saturated material used if drugs are otherwise unavailable.

Sativa Marihuana. From *Cannabis sativa*, the botanical name for the marihuana plant.

Saturday Night Habit Irregular use of small doses of narcotics.

Saturday Nighter Narcotics user who takes small doses at irregular intervals.

Sausage Marihuana.

Saxophone Opium pipe.

Scaffle PCP.

Scag Heroin.

Scales Weighing scales used to measure quantity of drug for sale.

Scar Heroin.

Scarf *Same as* Scroff.

Scars Black or blue areas of the skin resulting from narcotics injection.

Scat, Scatt Heroin.

Scene Place where something is happening, for example, where marihuana is being used.

Scheduled Drugs Drugs whose usage is restricted under the Drug Abuse Act of 1970.

Schlechts Narcotics. From Yiddish word meaning "bad."

Schlock Narcotics. From Yiddish word meaning "cheap merchandise."

Schmack *Same as* Schmeck.

Schmeck Heroin. From the German for "taste."

Schmecker Heroin user.

Schmeek *Same as* Schmeck.

Schnozzler Cocaine user. From *schnozzle*, meaning "nose."

Schoolboy Codeine.

Schroom Variant of mushroom, term for psilocybin.

Scissors Marihuana.

Scoff *Same as* Scroff.

Scoop 1. To sniff cocaine or heroin through a folded matchbook cover. 2. Folded matchbook cover through which cocaine or heroin is sniffed.

Scopolamine Psychoactive ingredient in *Datura*. Can cause hallucinations. Also produces relaxation and increased suggestibility. Used by police as "truth serum."

Score To locate and buy marihuana or any other drug.

Score Dough Money for narcotics.

Scott Heroin.

Scours Crude opium.

Scratching 1. Looking for drugs. 2. Behavior associated with early withdrawal from narcotics.

Scrip Prescription for narcotics.

Script *Abbreviation for* Prescription.

Script with a Tail *Same as* Reader with a Tail.

Scroff 1. To swallow a drug to avoid arrest. 2. To eat or swallow a drug rather than inject it.

Scuffle PCP.

Sealing Wax 1. Crude opium. 2. Hashish.

Sec Seconal, a barbiturate.

Seccies Seconal, a barbiturate.

Secobarbital sodium Short-acting barbiturate. Can cause physical and psychological dependence. Overdosage causes depression of central nervous system and respiratory arrest. Trade name is Seconal.

Seconal Secobarbital sodium, a barbiturate. Manufactured by Eli Lilly and Company. Comes in the form of red capsules.

Second Baseman The second person to smoke cocaine freebase at a party.

Secy, Seccy Seconal, a barbiturate.

Sedative Class of drugs that cause relaxation, calmness, and sedation in low doses and sleep in higher doses. Class includes barbiturates.

Seed Marihuana cigarette butt.

Seeds Morning-glory seeds.

Seeing Steve Using cocaine.

Seeing the Swing Man Meeting with a drug seller.

Seggy Seconal, a barbiturate.

Self-starter Narcotics user who voluntarily commits himself for treatment of his drug problem.

Send To smoke marihuana.

Send It Home To inject drugs intravenously.

Send Up Smoke Rings To smoke marihuana.

Seni Peyote.

Serendipity, Tranquility, Peace STP.

Serenity STP.

Sernyl Trade name for PCP.

Serotonin Neurochemical that modulates activity in the brain. Some drugs are believed to produce their effects by mimicking its actions.

Service Stripes Scars resulting from frequent intravenous narcotics injection.

Sess Sinsemilla.

Sessile Gland Gland in marihuana leaf that stores resin containing THC produced by trichomes.

Set 1. Expectations that affect reaction to drugs. Important only for very low doses. 2. Combination of Seconal, a barbiturate, and an amphetamine.

Set, Set of Works Paraphernalia for intravenous injection. *Same as* Artillery.

Set Me Straight Sell me drugs.

Set on His Ass Very intoxicated by a drug.

Setting Situation in which drug is taken. Can affect drug reaction especially for low doses of drugs.

Seven-foot Step Slow, gliding gait of person under the influence of marihuana.

Seven-one-fours (714s) Methaqualone.

Seventeen-fifty-one New York State drug law specifying minimum amount of drugs in one's possession for presumption of sale.

Sewer Vein into which narcotics are injected.

Shafer Commission National Commission on Marihuana and Drug Abuse headed by Chairman Raymond P. Shafer. The commission was appointed by President Nixon as part of the Comprehensive Drug Abuse Prevention and Control Act of 1970. The commission issued two reports: *Marihuana: Signal of Misunderstanding* (1972) and *Drug Use in America: Problem in Perspective* (1972).

Shake Resinous material that falls to bottom of sack during transit.

Shakedown 1. To search someone. 2. To try to get drugs regularly from a seller by telling him that narcotics have been hidden in the seller's room and that the narcotics police will be informed of it unless the seller cooperates.

Shaker Jar Vessel in cocaine kit for extracting cocaine freebase.

Sharp Euphoric as a result of taking a drug.

Sharps Hypodermic needles.

Shave 1. To adulterate a drug by adding inert material. 2. To use a razor blade to shave off a piece of morphine as it passes from dealer to dealer.

Sheets PCP.

Shermans PCP.

Sherms PCP.

Shishi Hashish.

Shit 1. Marihuana. 2. Heroin. 3. Demerol. 4. Dilaudid. 5. Any other "street drug."

Shlook Puff of marihuana smoke.

Shoot, Shoot Up 1. To inject a drug intravenously. 2. To take drugs successively for several hours.

Shoot below the Belt To inject narcotics in the hips or legs.

Shoot Gravy To inject the mixture of blood, water, and drug that may have cooled and coagulated if the initial injection could not be made due to a problem with the needle.

Shoot the Ack-Ack Gun To smoke heroin no. 3 off cigarettes in short, intense puffs. Term used primarily in Hong Kong.

Shoot Yen Shee To inject the opium residue from a Gee Rag.

Shooting Gallery Place where narcotics users congregate to inject themselves or be injected.

Shooting Gravy *See* Shoot Gravy.

Short 1. Loosely packed marihuana. 2. Quantity of drug that is less than paid for. 3. Brief sniff of a drug.

Short Connection Narcotics dealer who sells only small amounts.

Short Count Smaller amount of drug received than paid for.

Short Go Injection of small amount of narcotics.

Short Order *Same as* Short Go.

Short Piece Package of narcotics containing less drug than that paid for.

Shot Narcotics injection.

Shot in the Arm Narcotics injection into the arm.

Shot Put Injection of narcotics using a pin and an eye dropper.

Shot Up Under the influence of narcotics.

Shotgun 1. *Same as* Carburetor. 2. Guard who goes along with drug courier. 3. Brand name for amyl nitrite.

Shoulder Packing between needle and eye dropper used to inject narcotics.

Shove To sell narcotics.

Shovelling the Black Stuff Dependent on opium.

Shover Narcotics seller.

Shrooms Psilocybin.

Shuck To cheat, lie, deceive.

Shuzit Marihuana.

Shy To prepare opium for smoking.

Sick In need of narcotics to prevent further withdrawal.

Sickness Symptoms of withdrawal from narcotics.

Sifter Device for removing twigs and seeds from marihuana during cleaning.

Silk and Satin Combination of amphetamines and barbiturates.

Silly Putty Psilocybin.

Single Marihuana cigarette.

Single Convention United Nations agreement to limit exclusively to medical and scientific purposes the production, manufacture, export, import, distribution, use, and possession of certain drugs. The Single Convention was ratified by the United States in 1967.

Sinsemilla Spanish word meaning "without seeds"; marihuana made from unpollinated female marihuana flowers. Potent. Sinsemilla is produced by separating male plants from females before latter can be fertilized.

Sipping Smoking marihuana.

Sissy Cure Breaking the narcotics habit by gradually reducing the dosage over a period of time.

Sister Morphine.

Sitter *Same as* Babysitter.

Siva Hindu god. Revered because he was said to have swallowed poison from the sea that otherwise would have destroyed mankind. *Bhang* (marihuana) is taken as part of a religious devotion to Siva since Hindus believe he is very fond of it. Siva is known as the Lord of Bhang because he is believed to have brought bhang from the Himalayas for his devotees.

Sixteenth One-sixteenth of an ounce of diluted heroin.

Sizzle Narcotics in one's direct possession.

Skag Heroin.

Skamas Opium.

Skee Opium.

Skid Heroin.

Skid Bag Container of heroin.

Skid Row District in city where drunken derelicts congregate.

Skin Marihuana cigarette paper.

Skin Pop, Skin Popping Subcutaneous injection of drugs.

Skin Pumping *Same as* Skin Pop, Skin Popping.

Skinning *Same as* Skin Pop, Skin Popping.

Skinny 1. Marihuana cigarette paper. 2. Thin marihuana cigarette.

Skoofer Marihuana cigarette.

Skoofus Marihuana cigarette.

Skot Heroin.

Skrufer Marihuana cigarette.

Skrufus Marihuana cigarette.

Skuffle PCP.

Sky Rockets Amphetamines.

Slack-off Cure Breaking the narcotics habit by gradually reducing the dosage over a period of time.

Slag Heroin.

Slammer Jail.

Slap It Around To spread the good news.

Slapping the Bamboo Smoking opium.

Slave Master Water pipe for smoking marihuana.

Sleeper Heroin.

Sleepers Barbiturates.

Sleeping Pills Barbiturates.

Sleepwalker Heroin user.

Sleigh Riding Under the influence of narcotics.

Slumber Party Morphine.

Smack, Smak Heroin.

Smack Head Heroin user.

Smack-sack Heroin user.

Small Fry Drug seller with only a few customers as compared to more successful drug supplier who sells to dealers.

Small Stuff Drugs that do not cause physical dependence.

Smash Hash oil.

Smears LSD.

Smeck *Same as* Schmeck.

Smoke Marihuana.

Smokey Opium smoker.

Smoking PCP.

Smoking the Pipe Smoking opium.

Snake Marihuana smoker.

Snaker Chronic opium smoker.

Snap Amyl nitrite.

Snapper Amyl nitrite in a glass vial. From the opening or "snapping" of the vial so that the contents can be easily and quickly inhaled.

Snatch and Grab Junkie Narcotics user who also sells small amounts of heroin.

Sneaky Peat Marihuana mixed with wine.

Sneeze, Sneeze Down To detain a narcotics user without arresting him so that he may become an informer as his need for a drug increases.

Sneeze a Good Idea Where can I get cocaine?

Sneeze It Out To withdraw abruptly from narcotics. From the violent sneezing that accompanies withdrawal.

Sniff To inhale cocaine or heroin through the nose.

Sniffer Someone who sniffs cocaine or heroin.

Sniffing Inhaling cocaine or heroin through the nose.

Snoop Police officer.

Snop Marihuana.

Snort 1. Cocaine. 2. To sniff cocaine or heroin. 3. Drink of liquor. 4. PCP.

Snorter Paraphernalia item used for sniffing cocaine.

Snorting Sniffing a drug such as cocaine or heroin.

Snow 1. Cocaine. 2. Heroin. 3. Morphine.

Snow Ball Cocaine.

Snow Bird 1. Cocaine. 2. Morphine user.

Snow Caine Cocaine.

Snow Drifter Cocaine user.

Snow Flakes Cocaine.

Snow Flower Female cocaine user.

Snow Lights Visual hallucinations consisting of flickering white lights seen at the edges of the visual field. Associated with cocaine use.

Snow Shed Place where cocaine or other narcotics are hidden.

Snow Storm Hallucinations due to overdose of morphine.

Snowbase Use of nitrous oxide after smoking cocaine freebase.

Snowmobiling Taking cocaine.

Snozzle To sniff cocaine or heroin.

Soapers Methaqualone. From Sopor, a trade name for the drug.

Soaps Methaqualone. From Sopor, a trade name for the drug.

Sodium Base Cocaine freebase made with sodium hydroxide as solvent.

Soft Drug Term used to distinguish drugs such as marihuana, which do not cause physical dependence, from those such as heroin, which do cause physical dependence.

Softballs Barbiturates.

Sole Flat rectangular piece of hashish. So called because hashish smugglers in North Africa used them as false soles in their shoes to avoid detection by customs guards.

Solid Marihuana cigarette containing tobacco.

Solvent Volatile material containing hydrocarbons, such as glue, gasoline, and nail polish remover, which when inhaled cause initial stimulation and euphoria followed by stupor.

Soma 1. Mysterious drug mentioned in Hindu religious writings. Sometimes interpreted as reference to marihuana but usually as a reference to the mushroom *Amanita muscaria*. 2. PCP.

Somnos Trade name for chloral hydrate.

Son Lo Low-grade opium.

Son of One Hashish oil. Purer than previous distillates known as the One.

Sopes Methaqualone.

Sophisticated Lady Cocaine.

Sopor Methaqualone. Trade name used by Arnar-Stone Laboratories.

Soporific Producing sleep.

Sound Benactyzine hydrochloride.

Source Drug supplier of large quantities.

Space Cadet 1. Someone always intoxicated by drugs. 2. Burned out as a result of chronic drug use.

Spaced Out Dazed from drug use; disoriented; stuporous.

Spansula Combination of amphetamines and barbiturates.

Sparkle Plenties Amphetamines.

Sparklers Amphetamines.

Spear Hypodermic needle.

Special Potent marihuana cigarette.

Special Action Office for Drug Abuse Prevention (SAODAP) Federal agency established in 1972 to review all government agencies involved in drug abuse and to establish policies regarding drug abuse.

Speckled Birds Amphetamines.

Speed Amphetamines; usually used in reference to Methedrine.

Speed Demon *Same as* Speed Freak.

Speed Freak Frequent user of amphetamines.

Speed Palace Party at which methamphetamines are used.

Speedball 1. Combination of heroin and cocaine. 2. Combination of heroin and amphetamine. 3. Combination of Percodan and methamphetamine. 4. Combination of Dilaudid and cocaine.

Speeder Methamphetamine user.

Speeding 1. Using methamphetamines. 2 Drug-related stimulation.

Spike 1. Hypodermic needle. 2. Tobacco cigarette to which marihuana has been added.

Spike and Dripper Hypodermic needle and syringe.

Spike and Jolt Hypodermic needle and syringe.

Spiked Drug to which another drug has been added.

Spit Ball Exhaled cocaine freebase blown into someone's mouth. *Same as* Kiss.

Splach 1. Amphetamines. 2. To inject drugs intravenously.

Splash 1. Amphetamines. 2. To inject drugs intravenously.

Spliff Marihuana cigarette.

Splim Marihuana cigarette.

Splint Marihuana cigarette.

Split To leave, depart.

Splivins Amphetamines.

Spoon 1. Part of paraphernalia used to prepare heroin for injection. Handle is often twisted to make a loop through which a finger can be inserted to get a firm grip. Contents of spoon are heated so that heroin powder will dissolve in water. 2. Amount of amphetamine or other drug.

Spores PCP.

Sport of Gods Sniffing cocaine.

Spot Someone who acts as a lookout while another takes narcotics.

Spread the Good News To offer a marihuana cigarette.

Spring To offer a marihuana cigarette.

Sputterer Person who has just started smoking opium and doesn't believe he will become dependent.

Square Conformist; nonuser of drugs.

Square Apple *Same as* Square.

Square John Tobacco cigarette.

Squirrel 1.To store large amount of marihuana in a hiding place. 2. LSD.

S.S. Skin shot. Subcutaneous injection of drugs.

Stabber Safety pin used to pierce a vein to permit entry of eye dropper containing narcotics.

Stache Hidden supply of drugs.

Stack Quantity of marihuana cigarettes.

Star Dust 1. Cocaine. 2. PCP.

Stash *Same as* Stache.

Stash Container Paraphernalia item. Container for storing drugs.

Station Worker Narcotics user who injects drug rather than taking it orally.

Steam Roller Empty toilet tissue roll used as Steamboat.

Steamboat Empty box, tube, or rolled paper, with a hole for marihuana cigarette. Its purpose is to keep smoke from dissipating so that more can be inhaled.

Steel and Concrete Cure Sudden, forced abstinence from narcotics.

Steel Cure *Same as* Steel and Concrete Cure.

Steerer One who directs customers to a heroin seller in return for money or drugs from seller.

Stein Opium pipe.

Stella Brand of marihuana cigarette paper.

Stem Opium pipe.

Stem Artist Opium smoker.

Stencil Long, thin marihuana cigarette.

Stepped On Adulterated.

Stepping-Stone Theory Theory that marihuana use leads to use of other drugs.

Stick 1. Marihuana cigarette. 2. PCP.

Stimulants Class of drugs that cause increased brain activity resulting in sensation of greater energy, more alertness, and euphoria.

Sting To cheat.

Stinkweed 1. Marihuana. 2. Jimsonweed.

Stogie Thick marihuana cigarette.

Stomach Habit Taking drugs by mouth rather than by injection.

Stoned Very intoxicated by a drug to the point of immobility.

Stoner Narcotics user.

Stool Pigeon, Stoolie Informer.

Stool Pigeon Eyes Pupillary changes resulting from narcotics use.

Stoppers Barbiturates.

STP Dimethoxymethamphetamine (DOM). *STP* is abbreviation for "serendipity, tranquility, peace." Long-lasting hallucinogen, related in its chemical structure to amphetamine and mescaline.

Straight 1. Non–drug user. 2. Not under the influence of drugs. 3. Under the influence of marihuana. 4. Tobacco cigarette.

Straighten Out To smoke marihuana.

Straw Marihuana.

Strawberries 1. Amphetamines. 2. LSD.

Strawberry Fields LSD.

Street Dealer 1. Heroin seller who deals in small quantities. Buys from dealer in weight and sells to juggler. 2. Marihuana seller who deals in small quantities.

Street Drug Drug manufactured by a pharmaceutical company and diverted to illicit use, or used in a non–medically authorized way, or manufactured by an illegal laboratory.

Stretch To dilute a drug, for example, mixing oregano with marihuana.

Stretcher A substance used as an adulterant.

Strung (Out) 1. Dazed, disoriented, exhausted from drug use. 2. Using drugs heavily.

Student Inexperienced drug user.

Stuff Any drug.

Stuka Methamphetamine.

Stum Abbreviation for Stumblers.

Stumblers Barbiturates.

Subcutaneous Beneath the skin.

Substitutes Counterfeit drugs.

Suck Bamboo To smoke opium.

Sucker Weed Poor-quality or bogus marihuana.

Sudden Sniffing Death Syndrome Death caused by sniffing fluorocarbons contained in aerosols.

Suey Liquid solution made from the residue left in an opium pipe.

Suey Bowel Opium den.

Suey Pow Moistened sponge or rag used to wipe and cool opium bowl when cooking opium for smoking.

Sugar 1. Cocaine. 2. LSD. 3. Heroin. 4. Morphine.

Sugar and Salt Narcotics.

Sugar Con Confidence game in which buyer is sold narcotics, after which members of gang appear as police officers and arrest all. On the way to police station, bribery is suggested and accepted by fake police who confiscate drugs and all the money and leave.

Sugar Cube LSD. From the practice of placing a drop of the drug on a sugar cube for transport.

Sugar Lumps *Same as* Sugar Cube.

Sugar Weed *Same as* Sugared.

Sugared Marihuana soaked in sugared water and then dried. Purpose is to increase its apparent weight.

Summer Skies Morning-glory seeds.

Sun in the Moons Narcotics user who has just taken his drug.

Sunshine LSD.

Super PCP.

Super Blow Cocaine.

Super C Ketamine.

Super Charged 1. Drunk. 2. Intoxicated by a drug.

Super Dope Marihuana to which formaldehyde has been added.

Super Grass 1. Marihuana to which PCP has been added. 2. Ketamine.

Super Joint Marihuana cigarette to which PCP has been added.

Super Kools Marihuana to which PCP has been added.

Super Pot Marihuana soaked in alcohol and then dried.

Super Quaaludes Methaqualone.

Super Soper Methaqualone.

Super Weed Marihuana sprinkled with PCP.

Supercaine Substitute cocaine, usually lidocaine.

Superior Caine *Same as* Supercaine.

Supplier Drug seller.

Supremo Exceptionally high potency marihuana or hashish.

Surfer PCP.

Sweat It Out To undergo withdrawal from narcotics.

Sweat Room Place where narcotics user undergoes withdrawal.

Sweep To inhale cocaine.

Sweep with Both Barrels *Same as* Sweep.

Sweet Amphetamine capsule.

Sweet Jesus Morphine.

Sweet Lucy Marihuana soaked or extracted in wine.

Sweet Lunch Marihuana.

Sweet Morpheus Morphine.

Sweet Stuff Cocaine.

Sweets Amphetamines.

Swing into High Gear To become intoxicated by a drug.

Swing Man Drug seller.

Swinger Someone who uses many different drugs.

Swinging Uninhibited.

Swiss Purple High-quality LSD.

Sympathomimetic amines Substances that produce effects similar to those produced by ephinephrine.

Synanon Therapeutic community for rehabilitation of narcotics users. Established in 1959 in California.

Synergism Combined effect of two or more drugs such that the combination produces a greater effect than either alone. *See also* Additive effect; *same as* Potentiation.

Synesthesia Perception of sensations not normally associated with a stimulus, for example, hearing colors, seeing music.

Synhexyl Synthetic marihuanalike compound developed and used in 1940s on an experimental basis to treat depression.

Synthetic Acid STP.

Synthetic Cocaine PCP.

Synthetic Marihuana 1. THC. 2. Misnomer for PCP.

Synthetic narcotic, Synthetic opiate Drug that resembles morphine in effects, synthesized in the laboratory.

Synthetic THC PCP.

Syrup Dark brown heroin from Mexico.

T

T 1. *Abbreviation for* Tea. 2. PCP.

Tab Morphine.

Tabbing Placing a drop of LSD on a piece of paper.

Tabs 1. LSD. 2. Methamphetamine. 3. Any drug in tablet form.

Tac PCP.

Take a Pop To receive an injection of narcotics.

Take a Sweep To inhale drugs.

Take Off To rob.

Take the Boil-out To undergo withdrawal from narcotics.

Take the Cure To volunteer to undergo withdrawal from narcotics.

Take-off Artist Narcotics user who robs other drug users.

Taking Care of Business 1. Doing what has to be done to live. 2. Engaging in activities to get money to buy drugs.

Talk Down To reassure; calm; alleviate someone's drug-induced anxiety.

Tall Euphoric as a result of drug use.

Talwin Trade name for pentazocine hydrochloride. *See also* Ts and Blues.

Tambourine Man Drug seller.

Tap the Bag 1. To remove a small amount of heroin from its bag container before selling it. 2. To adulterate heroin.

Taper-off Cure Breaking the narcotics habit by gradually reducing the dosage over a period of time.

Tar Crude opium.

Tar Distiller Opium smoker.

Taste To try a sample of a drug before buying it to determine potency and general quality.

Taste Blood To begin narcotics use.

Taste Face Individual who loans his heroin paraphernalia in return for money or small supply of drug.

T-buzz PCP.

TCP Analog of PCP. Chemical name is 1-(1-[2-thienyl]cyclohexyl) piperidine hydrochloride.

Tea 1. Marihuana. Possibly from the fact that shredded marihuana looks like loose tea leaves, or because marihuana is "sipped," or because tea is sometimes brewed with marihuana. 2. PCP.

Tea Bag Marihuana cigarette.

Tea Blower Marihuana smoker.

Tea Head Marihuana smoker.

Tea Hound Marihuana smoker.

Tea Pad Place where marihuana is smoked.

Tea Party Gathering at which marihuana is smoked. Now called pot party.

Tea Shades Dark glasses worn by marihuana smokers.

Tead Up Under the influence of marihuana.

Tea-man 1. Marihuana smoker. 2. Marihuana seller.

Tecaba Heroin.

Tecato Narcotics user.

Teddies and Betties *Same as* Ts and Blues.

Teddy Party Marihuana.

Teenybopper Ten- to fifteen-year-old girl.

Temperature, Have a To be mildly intoxicated by a drug.

Temple Balls Balls of Nepalese hashish allegedly dried for seven years by Hindu holy men for later use in religious ceremonies. Now sold commercially.

Temple Bells *Same as* Temple Balls.

Temple Hash *Same as* Temple Balls.

Ten-cent Pistol Bag of "heroin" which instead contains poison.

Tens Amphetamines in 10-milligram dose.

Teo Marihuana smoker.

Tester Individual, usually heroin addict, who tests heroin for purity for dealer.

Tetrahydrocannabinol *See* THC.

Texas Leaguer Marihuana smoker.

Texas Tea Marihuana.

Thai Sticks Marihuana from Thailand. So called because it is formed from tops of marihuana plants wound around sticks of bamboo which are then bound together. Very potent and expensive.

THC 1. Tetrahydrocannabinol. The principal psychoactive ingredient in marihuana. 2. PCP misrepresented as THC either to deceive the buyer or because the effects are associated with THC.

THC Tabs PCP.

Thai Weed Marihuana from Thailand.

Therapeutic community Drug treatment program involving individual changes brought about through communal living. Method used by Synanon and other treatment centers.

Therapeutic dose Amount of drug required to produce an intended medical effect.

Therapeutic index Ratio between the therapeutic dose and the lethal dose.

There Intoxicated by marihuana.

Thin Hips Small hips from lying on one's side to smoke opium.

Thing 1. Marihuana cigarette. 2. Heroin.

Thiopental sodium Very short-acting barbiturate. Trade name is Pentothal.

Thirteen Marihuana cigarette. From the thirteenth letter of the alphabet, *M*.

Three-Day Habit Without narcotics for two to three days and beginning to feel acute withdrawal.

Thrill Pills Barbiturates.

Thriller Marihuana cigarette.

Through the Ceiling Very intoxicated by a drug.

Throw a Meter *See* Meter.

Throw Me Out With Give me a marihuana cigarette.

Thrusters Amphetamines.

Thumb Fat marihuana cigarette.

Thunder Weed Marihuana.

TIC PCP. From THC, the term given to PCP when it initially appeared.

Ticket Paper or blotter containing LSD.

Tic-tac PCP.

Tie Object used as a tourniquet to distend a vein for narcotics injection.

Tie Off To tie something tightly around the arm so that a vein will become prominent and easier to inject drugs into.

Tighten Up To smoke marihuana.

Tighten Your Wig To smoke marihuana.

Tin Container of marihuana.

Tin Action Purchase of tin of marihuana.

Tincture Drug preparation in which drug is dissolved in alcohol.

Tingle Initial effects of heroin felt in the chest.

Tinik Heroin.

Titch PCP. *See* TIC.

Tlitiltzen Morning-glory seeds.

TMA Trimethoxyamphetamine, a hallucinogen.

T-man 1. Federal narcotics agent, short for Treasury Man. The Treasury Department was responsible for narcotics control until 1968, when narcotics control was placed under the Justice Department. 2. Marihuana smoker.

TNT Heroin.

Toak, Toat *Same as* Toke.

Toilet Water Brand name for amyl nitrite.

Toke To inhale marihuana smoke.

Toke Pipe Short-stemmed pipe for smoking marihuana.

Toke Up To light a marihuana cigarette.

Toker 1. Marihuana smoker. 2. Glass pipe for smoking marihuana.

Tolerance Adaptation of the body to the point where more of a given drug is required to produce the same intensity of experience as that felt when first using it.

Toluene Volatile inhalant present in many industrial products such as glue.

Tooies 1. Barbiturates. 2. Tuinal capsules.

Tooles Barbiturates.

Tools Paraphernalia for intravenous injection. *Same as* Artillery.

Toot 1. Small amount of drug offered to the buyer to sample for quality. 2. Cocaine. 3. To sniff a drug.

Tootonium Expensive cocaine.

Toothpick Thin marihuana cigarette.

Tootsie Tuinal.

Top 1. Brand of marihuana cigarette paper—pot spelled backward. 2. Peyote.

Topi 1. Mescaline. 2. Peyote.

Tops Peyote.

Tops and Bottoms *See* Ts and Blues.

Torch 1. Marihuana cigarette. 2. Source of heat for smoking cocaine.

Torch Up To light a marihuana cigarette.

Torn Up Intoxicated by a drug.

Torpedo 1. Thick marihuana cigarette. 2. Whiskey to which chloral hydrate has been added.

Tossed Searched.

Totaled Physically and psychologically exhausted after an acute but intense drug experience.

Tote *Same as* Toke.

Tour Guide *Same as* Babysitter.

Toy Small opium container.

Tracks Scars resulting from frequent intravenous injection of narcotics.

Trafficker Drug seller.

Trafficking Selling drugs in large amounts. Usually used in reference to smuggling across borders.

Trank PCP.

Tranquilizers Drugs that have a calming, relaxing effect. Two main types are antianxiety tranquilizers and antipsychotic tranquilizers.

Travel Agent 1. LSD. 2. LSD seller. 3. *Same as* Babysitter.

Traveller One who uses hallucinogens.

Treat a J To add other drugs to a marihuana cigarette.

Treatment Alternatives to Street Crimes Federally sponsored program in which drug users who are arrested can enter a drug treatment program instead of going to jail.

Trees Tuinal capsules.

Tribed Up Full of narcotics.

Trichloracetaldehyde Chloral hydrate.

Trick Bag Diluted dose of drug.

Trigger To smoke marihuana after taking LSD.

Trip 1. Experience resulting from use of hallucinogens or marihuana. 2. To use hallucinogens.

Trip Grass Marihuana to which amphetamine has been added.

Trip Weed Marihuana.

Tripper One who uses hallucinogens.

Trips LSD.

Trolley Secret distribution pathways for narcotics.

Truck Drivers Amphetamines. From their use by long-distance truck drivers.

Ts and Blues Combination of Talwin (pentazocine) and Pyribenzamine (tripenelamine). Name is derived from Talwin trade name and blue color of Pyribenzamine. Talwin is an analgesic; pyribenzamine is an antihistamine. When combined and injected intravenously, the mixture is reputed to produce a heroinlike sensation.

T-Tabs PCP.

T-timers Dark glasses worn by marihuana smokers.

TT–1 PCP.

TT–2 PCP.

TT–3 PCP.

Tuck and Roll To fold ends of marihuana cigarette instead of twisting them.

Tuies Tuinal.

Tuinal Barbiturate containing amobarbital and secobarbital. Manufactured by Eli Lilly and Company. Comes in orange-and-blue capsule.

Tuned In Aware; involved; knowledgeable.

Turkey 1. To inhale marihuana smoke through the nose. 2. Amphetamines. 3 Cocaine. 4. Bogus drugs.

Turkey Trots Scars resulting from frequent intravenous injection.

Turn a Cartwheel To feign withdrawal in hopes of convincing a physician to administer or prescribe narcotics.

Turn On 1. To initiate someone into drug use. 2. To take a drug. 3. To give a drug as a gift.

Turn On, Tune In, Drop Out Slogan of hippie "flower children" of the 1960s, meaning "take drugs, become aware, renounce the materialistic world."

Turnabouts Amphetamines.

Turned On Under the influence of a drug.

Turnip Greens Marihuana.

Tuskee Thick marihuana cigarette.

Twenty-five LSD.

Twig Marihuana.

Twist Marihuana cigarette. From the twisted ends of marihuana cigarette, needed to keep the loose material from falling out.

Twist a Dream To roll a marihuana cigarette.

Twist a Giraffe's Tail To smoke marihuana.

Twist Scanner Marihuana user who makes new marihuana cigarettes out of butts.

Twisted Experiencing distress during withdrawal.

Twister Marihuana smoker.

Twisting a Few Smoking opium.

Two-arm Habit Narcotics user satisfied by injection into both arms.

Two-dollar Flop Visit to an opium den.

Two-toke Marihuana that can produce intoxication after just two inhalations.

Tying Up Placing a tourniquet around the arm for intravenous narcotics injection.

U

Uhffi Morphine.

Ultracaine Substitute cocaine, usually lidocaine.

Uncle 1. Federal narcotics officer. 2. Morphine.

Uniform Controlled Substances Act *See* Controlled Substances Act.

Uniform Drug Act Law developed by Federal Bureau of Narcotics in 1932 to make state drug laws compatible with federal laws.

Uniperversity College graduate who is dependent on narcotics.

Unkie Morphine.

Unkle 1. Morphine. 2. Federal narcotics agent.

Up Intoxicated; exhilarated.

Up against It Dependent on drugs.

Up and Down the Veins Repeated intravenous injections resulting in abscesses or collapsed veins that make location of veins for subsequent injection difficult.

Up and Up To stop using narcotics.

Up Quaalude Cocaine freebase. From dual sensation of stimulation and relaxation.

Uppers Amphetamines.

Uppie Amphetamines.

Ups Amphetamines.

Ups and Downs Amphetamines and barbiturates.

Uptight Nervous; anxious; tense.

Uptown Cocaine.

User Drug user.

Using Taking narcotics.

V

V Valium, an antianxiety tranquilizer. The most-prescribed drug in the United States.

Valley Crease above the elbow where the upper and lower arm meet. A favorite site for narcotics injection.

Vegged Out *Same as* Burned Out.

Vein Shooter Narcotics user who injects drug intravenously.

Vein Shot Intravenous injection of drugs.

Verification Shot Intravenous injection of narcotics wherein blood is drawn back into the syringe to make sure the needle is in the vein.

Veronal Trade name for barbital, one of the first barbiturates to be introduced in medicine.

Vials LSD.

Vibes Vibrations; feelings concerning someone or something.

Vipe To smoke marihuana.

Viper Marihuana smoker. Term imposed by marihuana users on themselves in the 1930s. Possibly originating from term "snake (viper) in the grass."

Viper Song Song about marihuana, for example, "Song of the Vipers."

Viperish Fond of marihuana.

Viper's Weed Marihuana.

Vonce Marihuana butt.

Voyager Someone on a "trip"; experiencing the effects of a hallucinogen.

V.S. *Abbreviation for* Vein Shot.

Vulture on the Veins Dependent on narcotics.

W

Wack To adulterate a drug by adding inert material.

Wacky Tobaccy Marihuana.

Wacky Weed, Whacky Weed Potent marihuana from Colombia, black in color.

Wafers Methadone.

Wahegan Potent marihuana from Hawaii.

Wake Up First injection of narcotics of the day.

Wake Ups Amphetamines.

Wakowi 1. Mescaline. 2. Peyote.

Walking on Air Intoxicated by a drug.

Wallbangers Methaqualone.

Wana Marihuana.

Waste 1. To smoke completely. 2. To kill.

Wasted Very intoxicated by a drug to the point of lethargy.

Water 1. Amphetamines. 2. PCP.

Water of Life Narcotics.

Water Pipe Pipe in which smoke is drawn through water to cool it and remove impurities.

Way Down 1. Needing marihuana. 2. Depressed because effects of drug have worn off.

Wedding Bells 1. Morning-glory seeds. 2. LSD.

Wedding Bells Acid LSD.

Wedges LSD.

Weed 1. Marihuana. 2. Misnomer for PCP.

Weed Eater Marihuana smoker.

Weed Head Marihuana smoker.

Weed Hound Marihuana smoker.

Weed Twister Marihuana smoker.

Weeding Out Smoking marihuana.

Weedly Female marihuana user.

Weekend Doper Casual drug user.

Weekend Habit *Same as* Weekend Doper.

Weekend Twister *Same as* Weekend Doper.

Weekend Warrior *Same as* Weekend Doper.

West Coast Turnabouts Amphetamines.

Whack Wack PCP.

Whack *Same as* Wack.

Whacky Tobacky *Same as* Wacky Tobacky.

Wheat Marihuana.

Where's Mary? Where can I get marihuana?

Whipped Cream Use of nitrous oxide after smoking cocaine free-base.

Whippets Nitrous oxide.

Whips and Jingles Early stages of withdrawal from narcotics.

Whiskers Police.

White Cocaine.

White Angel Morphine.

White Boy Heroin.

White Cross 1. Cocaine. 2. Amphetamines. 3. Heroin. 4. Morphine.

White Death 1. Cocaine. 2. Heroin. 3. Morphine.

White Dragon Pearl Heroin no. 3 combined with barbiturate and smoked in a cigarette.

White Girl Cocaine.

White Goddess Morphine.

White Horse Cocaine.

White Junk Heroin.

White Lady Cocaine.

White Linen Morphine.

White Lightning 1. Potent homemade whiskey. 2. LSD.

White Merchandise Morphine.

White Mosquito Cocaine.

White Nurse 1. Heroin. 2. Morphine.

White Owsley's LSD.

White Paste Coca paste.

White Powder 1. Cocaine. 2. PCP. 3. Heroin. 4. Morphine.

White Sandoz LSD.

White Silk Morphine.

White Stuff 1. Heroin. 2. Morphine. 3. Any drug that can be injected.

White Tape 1. Cocaine. 2. Morphine. 3. Heroin.

White Tornado Cocaine freebase.

Whites Amphetamines.

Whiz Bang 1. Mixture of heroin and cocaine. 2. Mixture of morphine and cocaine.

Who's Holding? Who has drugs for sale?

Wig Mind.

Wigged (Out) Loss of self-control.

Wild Geronimo Mixture of barbiturates and alcohol.

Wild Weed Marihuana growing wild; generally of low potency.

Windowpane LSD drop on cellophane or clear plastic.

Wing Ding To feign withdrawal in hopes of convincing a physician to administer or prescribe narcotics.

Wings 1. Cocaine. 2. Heroin. 3. Morphine.

Winky Pipe for smoking cocaine freebase.

Wiped Out Very intoxicated.

Wire Jail inmate who smuggles drugs to other inmates.

Wired Intoxicated by a drug.

Witch 1. Cocaine. 2. Heroin. 3. Morphine.

Witch Hazel Heroin.

Witch's Brew Combination of LSD and belladonna.

Withdrawal Various physical effects associated with cessation from chronic drug use. Withdrawal from narcotics results in influenzalike symptoms such as sweating, diarrhea, fever, and runny nose. In addition, yawning, dilation of pupils, rapid heart rate, and insomnia occur. Psychological reactions include hallucinations and delusions.

Wobble Weed PCP.

Wobbler To feign withdrawal in hopes of convincing a physician to administer or prescribe narcotics.

Wolf PCP.

Wooten Report British commission (1968) headed by Baroness Wooten that studied the effects of marihuana. The committee con-
cluded that marihuana was a relatively benign drug and recommended decriminalization and recognition that marihuana had
legitimate medical uses.

Works Paraphernalia for intravenous injection. *Same as* Artillery.

Worm PCP.

Wormy Experiencing onset of withdrawal from narcotics.

Wrecked *Same as* Wasted.

Y

Yale Hypodermic syringe. From the brand name.

Yellow Angel Nembutal, the barbiturate pentobarbital.

Yellow Birds Nembutal, the barbiturate pentobarbital.

Yellow Bullets Nembutal, the barbiturate pentobarbital.

Yellow Dimples LSD.

Yellow Fever 1. LSD. 2. PCP.

Yellow Jackets Nembutal, the barbiturate pentobarbital.

Yellow Sunshine LSD.

Yellows 1. Nembutal, the barbiturate pentobarbital. From color of capsule. 2. LSD.

Yen 1. Craving for narcotics. 2. Opium.

Yen Chee Opium pellet.

Yen Chiang Opium pipe.

Yen Gow Steel tool used by opium cooks to cleanse and scrape ashes from opium pipe bowl.

Yen Hock, Yen Hoke Thin steel rod on which opium pill is cooked before it is placed in bowl to smoke.

Yen in the Cheek Green opium placed in the back of lower teeth.

Yen On Narcotics withdrawal.

Yen Pock Cooked opium that is eaten.

Yen Pook Small, cooked opium pill.

Yen Shee Charred opium ashes scraped from opium pipebowl and often eaten or dissolved in water and injected.

Yen Shee Baby Hard stools associated with constipation caused by opium.

Yen Shee Boy Opium user.

Yen Shee Gow Steel tool used by opium cooks to cleanse and scrape ashes from opium pipe bowl. *Same as* Yen Gow.

Yen Shee Quay Opium user.

Yen Shee Suey Opium solution.

Yen Yen Relaxation from smoking opium.

Yenning Experiencing withdrawal from narcotics.

Yerba Marihuana. From Spanish *herba* meaning "weed."

Yesca Marihuana.

Youngblood Beginning marihuana smoker.

Yummies Any drug.

Z

Z Ounce of drug.

Zacatecas Purple Potent marihuana from Mexico.

Zen LSD.

Zig-Zag Brand of marihuana cigarette paper.

Zig-Zag Man Man depicted on Zig-Zag paper.

Zipped Under the influence of a drug.

Z-kit Paraphernalia item consisting of marihuana pipe, roach clip, book of matches, and various other accessories.

Zol Marihuana cigarette. Term primarily used in South Africa.

Zombie Buzz Very potent PCP, brown in color.

Zombie Weed Marihuana to which PCP has been added.

Zonked Under the influence of a drug; so intoxicated that one is unaware of one's surroundings.

Zooie Cylindrical device for holding butt of marihuana cigarette.

Zoom Marihuana to which PCP has been added.

Glossary

Most of the terms listed in the glossary can be found in this dictionary.

Abstinence, drug: Away, Away from the Habit, Break the Habit, Break the Needle, Clean, Clean Head, Clean Up, Cleaned, Clear Up, Fold Up, Get the Monkey off My Back, Get the Vulture off My Veins, Go Straight, Goof Head, Kick the Habit, Mature, Out-of-it, Quitter, Shake the Habit, Straight, Up and Up. *See also* Addict, trying to quit habit; Withdrawal

Addict: Ad, Arctic Explorer, Bed Bugs, Bindle Bum, Bindle Stiff, Bowin, Chronic, D.A., Dip, Dope, Dope Fiend, Dope Head, Dope Hop, Doper, Dopester, Down to the Cotton, Dreamer, Dug Out, Feeblo, Fiend, Flier, Gargoyle, Geed, Glass Eyes, Glassy Eye, Gow Head, Gowster, Greasy Junkie, Habitué, Hag, Have On the Feed Bag, Hit the Hop, Hit the Stuff, Hop Hog, Hop Merchant, Hop Head, Hopster, Hype, Hype Shooter, Junk Hog, Junk Hound, Junk Man, Junker, Junkie, Junky, Knocker, Liner, Locust, Low Rider, Mount, Narco, Pasty Face, Pick Up, Pin Head, Roller, Slim, Smack Head, Smack-sack, Smecker, Snatch, Snatch and Grab Junkie, Stoner, Up against It. *See also* Narcotics user

Addict, former. *See* Addict, trying to quit habit

Addict, new. *See* Narcotics use, beginning

Addict, impoverished: Cotton Picker, Cotton Shooter, Down to the Cotton

Addict, by intravenous injection: Bangster, Channel Swimmer, Gutter, Hype, Hype Shooter, Hypo, Hypo Juggler, Hypo Smacker, Hypo Smecker, Jabber, Liner, Mainline Shooter, Mainliner, Needle Fiend, Needle Jabber, Needle Man, Needle Nipper, Needle Pusher, Needle Rusher, Vein Shooter, V.S. *See also* Injection, intravenous

Addict, irregular: Chipper, Chippy, Cotton Picker, Fortnightey, Joy Popper, Joy Rider, Kick Freak, Light-weight Chipper, Period Hitter, Pleasure User, Saturday Nighter, Weekend Doper, Weekend Twister, Weekend Warrior, Weekender. *See also* Irregular Drug Use

Addict, trying to quit habit: Dope Fighter, Knocker, Pug, Self-starter, Volunteer. *See also* Abstinence, drug

Addiction: Ad, Ad-it, Army Disease, Bamboozled, Be in Business, Be On, Betting on the Horse, Bindle Stiffened, Bite, Booking with Charlie, Bunk Habit, Casing the Nurse, Caught on the Needle, Chasing the Nurse, Chasing the White Nurse, Chew the Fat, Chinaman, Chinaman on (One's) Back, Chippy Habit, Coffee Habit, Cotton Habit, Courting Cecile, Dependence, Dipped, Eating Poppy Seed Cakes, From Mount Shasta, Gow Headed, Habit, Habituation, Have a Habit, Have a Yen, Have an Itch, Hit and Miss Habit, Hit by the Hop, Hit the Gow, Hit the Stuff, Hooked, Hop on the Monkey Wagon, Hung Out, Hung Up, Ice Cream Habit, Jockey, Kicked by a Horse, King Kong, Lamp Habit, Mixed in the Mud, Monkey Bite, Monkey in the Wool, Monkey on (One's) Back, Monkey Wagon, Mouth Habit, Narcotism, Narkied, On the Horse, On the Mojo, On the Needle, On the Pipe, On the Stuff, Pasted, Picking the Poppies, Poppy Headed, Riding the Poppy Train, Riding the Witch's Broom, Saturday Night Habit, Shovelling the Black Stuff, Strung (Out), Stuka, Stung by the Hop, Two-arm Habit, Up against It, Vulture on the Veins

Adulteration: Bonaroo, Bull Jive, Burned, Catnip, Chip, Cut, Dilutant, Doctor, Dust, Manita, Shave, Stepped On, Stretcher, Trick Bag, Wack

Aftereffect: Crash, Down, Dragged, Fall Out, Flake, Out, Rock Out

Amobarbital sodium. *See* Amytal sodium

Amphetamines: A, Aimies, Amp, Amt, Amy, B-29s, Bam, Bambita, Bams, Bean, Beans, Bennies, Benny, Benz, Benzedrine, Black Beauties, Black Bombers, Black Bottle, Blue Angel, Bombida, Bombido, Bombita, Bottles, Box of L, Brain Ticklers, Brownies, Browns, Bumble Bees, Businessman's Lunch, Cartwheels, Chalk, Christina, Christmas Tree, Coast-to-coasts, Co-pilot, Crank, Cranks, Crink, Cris, Cross Countries, Crossroads, Cross Tops, Crosses, Crystal, Desoxyn, Dex, Dexedrine, Dexies, Dexo, Dexy, Dominoes, Double cross, Drivers, Dynamite Stocks, Eye Opener, Fives, Football, Forwards, Glass, Goies, Grads, Green Dragon, Greenies, Hearts, Horse Heads, Inbetweens, Jam, Jam Cecil, Jelly Babies, Jelly Beans, Jolly Beans, Joy Pellet, L.A. Turnabouts, Leapers, Lid Poppers, Lightning, Lip Proppers, Meth, Methedrine, Minibennies, Nuggets, Orange, Peaches, Pep Pills, Pep-em-ups, Pixies, Powder, Purple Hearts, Roses, Rhythms, Rippers, Road Dope, Sky Rockets, Sparkle Plenties, Sparklers, Speckled Birds, Speed, Splach, Splash, Splivins, STP, Stuka, Sweet, Sweets, Tabs, Thrusters, TMA, Truck Drivers, Turnabouts, Uppers, Uppie, Ups, Wake-ups, Water, West Coast Turnabouts, Whites

Amphetamine user: A-head, Bean head, Benzadrina, Crank Commando, Hyper, Meth Freak, Meth Head, Meth Monster, Pill Head, Speed Demon, Speed Freak, Speeder

Amyl nitrite: Amy, Amy joy, Aroma of Man, Ban Apple, Black Jack, Bolt, Bullet, Cat's Meow, Cum, Dr. Bananas, Hardware, Heart On, Hi Baller, Jac Aroma, Loc-A-Roma, Locker Popper, Locker Room, Oz, Pearls, Poppers, Rush, Satan's Scent, Shotgun, Snappers, Sniffers, Toilet Water

Amytal Sodium: Amobarbital Sodium; Bands, Blue Angel, Blues, Blue Birds, Blue Bullets, Blue Clouds, Blue Devils, Blue Heavens, Blue Jackets, Blue Tips, Bullets, Devils. *See also* Barbiturates

Apprehension, due to drug use: Bull Horror, Horrors, Paranoia, Pig Rap

Arrest (law enforcement): Batted Out, Been Had, Busted, Bum Rap, Canned, Clipped, Collared, Cooler, Cop a Plea, Cop Out, Dope Lawyer, Dropped, Duke In, Federal Beef, Felony, Flag, Glued, Heat, Heat's On, Horrors, Hummer, Misdemeanor, Nicked, Nailed, On Ice, Operation Intercept, Paid Off in Gold, Plant, Popped, Violated. *See also* Inform

Barbiturates: Amies, Backwards, Bank Bandits, Barbs, Black Beauties, Black Mollies, Blockbusters, Blues, Blunt, Brain Ticklers, Candy, Christmas Roll, Courage Pills, Dolls, Gangster Pills, G.B., Goofballs, Goofers, Gorilla Pills, Green Dragon, Hexobarbital, Joy Pellets, King Kongs, King Kong Pills, Mighty Joe Young, Peanuts, Pills, Sleepers, Sleeping Pills, Softballs, Stum, Stumblers, Stuppers, Thrill Pills, Tooies, Tooles, Veronal. *See also* Amytal Sodium, Nembutal, Phenobarbital, Seconal, Tuinal

Chloral hydrate: Black Bottle, Coral, Gongo with a Jump, Heel Tap, Joy Juice, Keeler, Knockout Drops, Mickey Finn, Mickey Flynn, Noctec, Peter, Somnos, Trichloracetaldehyde

Cocaine: Baking Soda Base, Base, Bernice, Bernies, Bernie's Flake, Big Bloke, Big C, Billie Hoak, Birdie Powder, Blinky, Bounce Powder, Bouncing Powder, Brute, Burese, Burnies, C, Cabello, Cacil, Cadillac, Came, Candy Cee, Carrie, Carrie Nation, Cecil, C-duct, Cee, Chalk, Charley, Cheese, Chick, Cholly, C-jam, Coca, Coca Paste, Cocoanut, Cola, Cookie, Corine, Doctor White, Duct, Dust, Flake, Florida Snow, Foo Foo Dust, Foolish Powder, Freebase, Frisking Powder, Gin, Girl, Glad Stuff, Gold Dust, Golden Girl, Goofy Dust, Happy Dust, Heaven Dust, Her, Hocus, Ice, Incentive, Jam, Joy Dust, Joy Flakes, Joy Powder, Lady, Lady Snow, Lady White, Mayo, Med Mojo, Monkey Cocaine, Mosquito, Nose, Nose Candy, Nose Powder, Nose Stuff, Number Three, Old Madge, Old Slave, Paradise, Perico, Piece, Pimp Dust, Pogo Pogo, Poison, Powder, Powder Diamonds, Racehorse Charlie, Rane, Rock, Snort, Snow, Snow Ball, Snow Bird, Snow Caine, Snow Flakes, Sport of Gods, Sugar, Super Blow, Toot, Tootonium, Turkey, Uptown, White, White Cross, White Death, White Girl, White Horse, White Lady, White Mosquito, White Paste, White Powder, White Tape, White Tornado, Witch

Cocaine use: Base Binge, Base Dreams, Baseball, BBs, Billied, Blow, Blow Charlie, Blow Coke, Blow Snow, Caught in a Snow Storm, Cocaine Blues, Cocaine Bugs, Cocainized, Coke Bugs, Coked Out, Ear Rings, Feeding Candy, Get Your Nose Cold, Go on a Sleigh Ride, Horn, Kiss, Scoop, Seeing Steve, Sniff, Snort, Snowmobiling, Snozzle, Sweep with Both Barrels

Cocaine user: Artic Explorer, Baseman, Bloker, C-head, Candy Fiend, Candy Head, Charley Coke, Cocaine Anonymous, Cocainist, Coke Freak, Coke Head, Coke Whore, Cokey, Cokomo, First Baseman, Forty-niner, Horner, Kokomo, Kokomo Joe, Schnozzler, Sniffer, Snorter, Snow Drifter, Snow Flower

Codeine: Four-doors, Fours, Leads, MED, Methylmorphine, Robe, Schoolboy, Second Baseman, Third Baseman

Combination, amobarbital and secobarbital: Double Trouble, Rainbow, Reds and Blues, Tuinal

Combination, amphetamine and barbiturate: Bam, Black Widow, Bombita, Christmas Tree, Desbutyl, French Blue, Green Hornet, Greenies, Set, Silk and Satin, Spansula, Ups and Downs

Combination, cocaine and other drugs: C and H, C and M, Cannon Ball, Cod Cock, Coke and Crystal, Cold and Hot, Frisko Speedball, H and C, Love Affair, Marmon and Cadillac, Monroe in a Cadillac, Speedball, Whiz Bang

Combination, marihuana and other drugs: A-bomb, Atom Bomb, Banana with Cheese, Booster Stick, Camphor, Candy a Joint, Chicharra, Cocktail, Crystal Joint, Dust, Dust Joint, Heavy Joint, Lovely, Lusher, Mule, O.J., Opiated Hash, Rocket Fuel, Sneaky Peat, Solid, Spiked, Super Dope, Super Grass, Super Kools, Super Pot, Super Weed, Sweet Lucy, Treat a J, Trigger, Trip Grass, Zombie Weed, Zoom

Container, Drug: B, Bag, Baggie, Balloons, Feed Bag, Matchbox, Toy

Dilaudid: Juice, Little D, Lords, Shit

Doctor: Croaker, Dr. Feelgood, Ice Tong Doctor, Ice Water John, Right Croaker

Drug Buys. *See* Drugs, purchase and sale

Drug Commissions: Commission of Inquiry into the Nonmedical Use of Drugs, Indian Hemp Drug Commission, La Guardia Report, Le Dain Commission, LEMAR, Narcotic Addiction Control Commission, National Commission on Marihuana and Drug Abuse, Panama Canal Zone Military Inquiry, President Johnson's Commission on Law Enforcement and Administration of Justice, President Kennedy's Ad Hoc Panel on Drug Abuse, Wooten Report

Drug enforcement agencies: Bureau of Narcotics and Dangerous Drugs, Drug Enforcement Agency, Drug Policy Office, Federal Bureau of Narcotics

Drug Factory: Brewery, Feed Store, Kitchen Lab, Lab, Midnight Lab, Pig Outfit

Drug Manufacture: Capping, Dusting, Roll, Stretch

Drug Organizations: AA, Adamha, Addiction Research Foundation, Alliance for Cannabis Therapeutics, American Council on Marihuana and Other Psychoactive Drugs, Amorphia, Bureau of Narcotics and Dangerous Drugs, Center for Multicultural Awareness, Client Oriented Data Acquisition Process, Daycare, Daytop Village, Drug Abuse Council, Drug Abuse Warning Network, Federal Drug Abuse Policy, Halfway House, Lemar, Narconon, Narcotics Anonymous, Narcotics Treatment Administration, National Committee on the Treatment of Intractable Pain, National Drug Abuse Treatment Utilization Survey, National Institute on Drug Abuse, National Institute of Mental Health, National Institute on Alcohol Abuse and Alcoholism, National Organization for the Reform of Marihuana Laws, National Survey in Drug Abuse, Native American Church, Odyssey House, Office of Drug Abuse Law Enforcement, Special Action Office for Drug Abuse Prevention, Synanon.

Drug seller: Bag Man, Big Man, Broker, Candy Man, Connection, Connector, Contact, Cop Man, Cowboy, Dealer, Dope Peddler, Dope Pimp, Dope Runner, Drug Booster, Feed and Grain Man, Good Time Man, Grog Merchant, Ice Cream Man, Jobber, Junk Peddler, Junker, Live Bait, Man, Man from Montana, Margin Man, Missionary, Mother, Operator, Ounce Man, Panic Man, Paper Boy, Peddler, Pied Piper, Pusher, Righteous Dealer, Short Connection, Steerer, Street Dealer, Supplier, Swig Man, Tamborine Man, Thoroughbred, Trafficker, Travel Agent. *See also* Drugs, purchase and sale; Drug seller, dishonest

Drug seller, dishonest: Burn artist, Con, Coyote

Drugs, purchase and sale: Buzzing, Connect, Cop, Cop a Buy, Cop a Fix, Cop a Match, Deal, Deal in Weight, Deuce Someone, Freeze, Front, Get Through, Grass Action, Hit, In Front of the Gun, Junk Craft, Make a Buy, Make a Meet, Make the Man, Pick Up, Pound Action, Prime the Pump, Put Me Straight, Score, Short Count, Sneeze a Good Idea, Tin Action, Toot

Effects, of chronic drug use: Beaten, Brain Burned, Burned Out, Cut Off, Destroyed, Echoes, Flipped, Fried, Fucked Up, O.D., Ozoned, Strung Out, Totalled, Vegged Out, Wasted, Wigged Out, Wrecked. *See also* Exhaustion, due to drug use; Under the influence, of a drug

Effects, loss of: Bring Down, Cap Out, Come Down, Come Home, Fall Out

Exhaustion, due to drug use: Beaten, Destroyed, Spent, Vegged Out, Whipped, Wiped out

Experience, drug, unpleasant: Acid Funk, Bad Head, Bad Trip, Bum Bend, Bum Trip, Bummer, Crank Bugs, Dragged, Ear Rings, Flip, Freak Out, O.D., Panic Reaction, Way Down

Forensic test: Beam Test, Chromatograph, Dille-Koppanyi Test, Duquenois Test, False Negative, False Positive

Glue, sniffer/sniffing: Blowing the Bag, Flashing, Gassing, Gluey, Huffing, Rowdy

Hashish: Afghani, African Black, Bambalacha, Black, Black Hash, Black Russian, Blond, Blue Cheese, Candy, Charas, Chocolate, Chunk, Citroli, Dope Smoke, Green Moroccan, Hash, Heavy Hash, Heesh, Hog, Indian Rope, Leb, Lebanese, Lightening Hash, Mud, Nepalese Hash, Nepalese Temple Balls, Nepalese Temple Hash, Pakistani Hash, Powder, Quarter Moon, Red Lebanese, Sealing Wax, Shishi, Sole, Temple Balls, Temple Bells, Temple Hash. *See also* Hashish Oil

Hashish oil: Afghani, Black Oil, Cherry Leb, Honey Oil, Indian Oil, Oil, One, Red Oil, Smash, Son of One, The One. *See also* Hashish

Heroin: Ack Ack, Antifreeze, Aunt Hazel, Aunt Noral, Bad Bundle, Balot, Big Boy, Big H, Big Harry, Bonita, Boy, Bozo, Brown, Brown Rhine, Brown Rock, Brown Stuff, Brown Sugar, Caballo, Caca, China White, China White Goods, Chinese Red, Cobics, Corgy, Courage Pills, Crap, Crown Crap, Deck, Diacetylmorphine, Dog Food, Dogie, Dope, Downtown, Du-

gee, Dyno, Ferry Dust, Foolish Powder, Galloing Horse, Gammot, George
Smack, H, H-cap, Hairy, Halvah, Harry, Hazel, Henry, Hero, Heroin
No. 3, Heroin No. 4, Him, Hocus, Horse, Horse Radish, HRN, Isda, Jee
Gee, Jive Do Jee, Jones, Joy Dust, Joy Flakes, Joy Powder, Ka Ka, Ka-
bayo, Kenkoy, Matsakaw, Mayo, McCoy, Merchandise, Mexican Mud,
Monkey Heroin, Muscle, Oil, Old Steve, Oroy, Pack, Piece, Poison,
Powder, Pulborn, Pure, Rat Poison, Red Chicken, Red Rock, Rock, Salt,
Scag, Scar, Scat, Schlechts, Schlock, Schmack, Schmeck, Schmeek, Scott,
Shit, Skag, Skid, Skot, Slag, Sleeper, Smack, Smeck, Snow, Sugar, Syrup,
Tinik, TNT, White Dragon Pearl, White Nurse, White Powder, White
Stuff, White Tape, Witch, Witch Hazel. *See also* Narcotics

Hidden drugs: Arsenal, Asscache, Cache, Coozie Stash, Finger Wave, Snow
Shed, Stache, Stash. *See also* Smuggling

High: Belted, Bent, Bent Out of Shape, Blasted, Blitzed, Bombed, Boxed,
Charged, Coasting, Floating, Gassed, Grooving, Hopped, Jacked Up,
Loaded, Locked, Singing, Smashed, Spaced, Spiked, Stoned, Tall, Torn
Up, Twisted. *See also* Exhaustion, due to drug use

Hunger, associated with drug use: Chuck Habit, Chuck Horrors, Chuckers,
Hungries, Hungry Horrors

Inform: Burn, Blower, Cop, Duke in, Fagan, Finger, Fink, Flag, Long Tail Rat,
Louse, Mouse, Poison, Rat, Sting, Stool Pigeon, Stooly, Take off. *See also*
Arrest

Initial effects, drug injection: Charge, Flash, Jolt, Kick, Splash, Thrill, Tingle,
Zing. *See also* High

Injection, drug: Bang, Bing, Chicago Leprosy, Dead Bag, Fire Up, Fix, Jab,
Joy Pop, Joy Prick, Keek, Knife in the Arm, Mainline, Muscle, Ping in
the Wing, Pop, Prod, Prop, Shoot Below the Belt, Shoot Up, Shoot Yen
Shee, Skin Pop, Skin Pumping, Skinning, S.S., Take a Pop. *See also*
Injection, intravenous

Injection, intravenous: Back Up, Bang, Bang in the Arm, Banging, Booting,
Broach, Bust the Mainline, Cave, Cave Digging, Chinese Needle Work,
Crater, Cushion, Ditch, Do Up, Douche, Drop Shot, Drilling, Five,
Flushing, Gate, Geezing, Get with It, Getting Off, Give Wings, Go in
the Gutter, Gravy, Gutter, Hit the Sewer, Hitting, Hype, Jabbing, Jack,
Jacking Off the Spike, Jerk Off, Jolting, Laugh and Scratch, Line Shot,
Lining, Lip the Dripper, Mainlining, Monkey Doodle, Needle Happy,
Needle Sharing, Needle Shy, Needle Trouble, Needle Yen, Pen Shot,
Penitentiary Shot, Pipe, Pit, Pocks, Raise a Welt, Register, Roller, Scars,
Send it Home, Service Stripes, Sewer, Shoot Gravy, Shooting Gallery,
Shoot Up, Short Go, Short Order, Shot, Shot in the Arm, Shot Pin,
Splach, Splash, Tap, Tie Off, Tracks, Tracked, Turkey Trots, Tying Up,
Up and Down the Veins, Valley, Vein Shot, Verification Shot, V.S. *See
also* Addict, by intravenous injection

Intoxication, drug. *See* High; Under the influence, of a drug

Irregular drug use: Chicken Shit Habit, Chip, Chippy Habit, Dabble, Dabbling, Dip and Dab, Fortnightey, Hit and Miss Habit, Ice Cream Habit,

In the Chips, Joy Pop, Light-Weight Nothing, Live in the Suburbs, Mickey Mouse Habit, Play Around, Saturday Night Habit, Three Day Habit, Weekend Habit. *See also* Addict, irregular

Jail, Jailed: Boxed, Can, Federal Beef, Fin, Flat Time, Full Time, Hack, Hard Time, Iced, Iron House, Joint, Lock Up, Narco Rap, Nickel, Number Two Sale, On Ice, Slammed, Slammer

Ketamine: Jet, K, Super C

Legislation, drug: Ann Arbor Ordinance, Antiparaphernalia Law, Boggs Act, Comprehensive Drug Abuse Prevention and Control Act, Controlled Substance Act, Decriminalization, Drug Abuse Act of 1970, El Paso ordinance, Harrison Act, Marihuana and Health Reporting Act, Marihuana Tax Act, Narcotic Addiction Control Commission, Narcotic Addiction Rehabilitation Act of 1966, Narcotic Control Act, Narcotic Limitation Convention of 1931, Operation Intercept, Oregon Decriminalization Bill, Pure Food and Drug Act, Single Convention, Uniform Controlled Substances Act, Uniform Drug Act

Location, cocaine use: Coke Oven, Coke Party

Location, heroin use: Bang Room, Bing Room, Bingo Room, Dutch Mill, Old Lady's Place

Location, marihuana use: Balloon Room, Ballroom, Blast Party, Club, Crash Pad, Dopatorium, Dope Den, Doperie, Pot Party

Location, opium use: Black Spot, Brewery, Business, Fun Joint, Gonger Den, Joint, Lay, Opium Joint, Opiumery, Pipe Factory, Poppy Alley, Poppy Grove, Suey Bowl

Location, PCP use: Crystal Palace

LSD: A, Acid, Ad, Animal, Beast, Big D, Black Tabs, Blue Acid, Blue Chairs, Blue Cheers, Blue Flag, Blue Heaven, Blue Mist, Blue Owsley, Brown Dots, California Sunshine, Candy, Cherry Top, Chief, Coffee, Cracker, Cubes, Cupcakes, Deeda, Delysid, Domes, Dot, Flash, Flat Blues, Flats, Four Way Hit, Ghost, Grape Parfait, Green Dragon, Green Swirls, Green Wedge, Hawaiian Sunshine, Hawk, Haze, Insant Zen, L, LBJ, Lucy in the Sky with Diamonds, Mary Owsley, Microdots, Mighty Quinn, Mind Detergent, One Way Hit, Orange Cubes, Orange Micro, Orange Mushroom, Orange Owsley, Orange Sunshine, Orange Wedges, Outer, Owsley, Owsley's Aud, Owsley's Blue Dot, Peace, Peace Tablets, Pink Owsley, Pink Swirl, Pink Wedge, Pure Love, Purple Barrels, Purple Flats, Purple Haze, Purple Microdots, Purple Ozoline, Royal Blues, Sandoz, Squirrel, Strawberries, Strawberry Fields, Sugar, Sugar Cube, Sugar Lumps, Sunshine, Swiss Purple, Tabs, Travel Agent, Trips, Twenty-Five, Two Way Hit, Vials, Wedding Bells, Wedding Bells Acid, Wedges, White Lightning, White Owsley's, White Sandoz, Yellow Dimples, Yellow Fever, Yellow Sunshine, Yellows, Zen. *See also* LSD on paper

LSD on paper: Blotter, Blue Dot, Blue Splash, Contact Lens, Clear Light, D, Electric Kool Aid, Flake Acid, Gelatin, Love Saves, Paper, Raggedy-Ann, Ticket, Windowpane. *See also* LSD

LSD user: Acid Dropper, Acid Freak, Acid Head, Experimenter, Explorer's Club, Traveller

Marihuana: Ashes, Aunt Mary, Baby, Baby Buds, Bambalacha, Bang, Birdwood, Blue de Hue, Blue Sage, Bo Bo, Bo Bo Bush, Boo, Brifo, Broccoli, Bu, Budda, Buddha Sticks, Bush, Busy, Butter Flower, Cannabis, Canned Goods, Carmabus, Charge, Chiba Chiba, Chira, Churus, Dagga, Ding, Dona Juanita, Doobie, Dope, Dope Smoke, Dubie, Faggot, Fennel, Fu, Funny Stuff, Gage, Gangster, Ganja, Gash, Gates, Gauge, Gear, Giggle Smoke, Goof Butt, Grass, Greefa, Greefo, Green Griff, Grefa, Greta, Griefo, Grifa, Griffa, Grifo, Gunja, Gunjeh, Gunny, Happy Gas, Happy Grass, Hay, Hemp, Herb, HOG, Hooch, Hot Hay, Incense, Indian Bay, Indian Hay, Indian Hemp, Indian Weed, J Smoke, Jahooby, Jingo, Jive, Johnson, Joy Smoke, Ju Ju, Juane, Juanita, Juanita Weed, Kaif, Kanjac, Keef, Kheef, Kif, Laughing Grass, Laughing Tobacco, Leaves, Loco Weed, Love Weed, Lozies, Lozerose, M, Mach, Maggie, Mari, Mariahuana, Mary, Mary and Johnny, Mary Ann, Mary Anner, Mary Jane, Mary Juana, M.J., Mary Warner, Mary Weaver, Mary Werner, Megg, Mesca, Mex, Mexican, M.O, Modams, Mohasky, Mojo, Mooca, Mootah, Mooter, Mootie, Mor a Grifa, Motta, Mu, Mud, Murder Weed, Muta, Noble Weed, Pleiku Pink, Pod, Pot, Powder, Ragweed, Railroad Weed, Rangoon, Red, Red Dirt Marihuana, Red Gunyon, Reefer, Righteous Bush, Rocket, Sativa, Sausage, Shit, Shuzit, Smoke, Snop, Stinkweed, Straw, Stuff, Sweet Lunch, Sweet Mary, T, Tea, Texas Tea, Thunder Weed, Viper's Weed, Wacky Tobaccy, Weed, Wheat, Yerba, Yesca, Zoom. *See also* Hashish
Marihuana, domestic: Bethesda Gold, Black Columbus, Breckenridge Green, Chicago Black, Chicago Green, Columbus Black, Gainesville Green, Home-grown, Jersey Green, Kentucky Blue, Manhattan Silver, Manhattan White, New York White, Tennessee Blue, Wahegan, Wild Weed
Marihuana, foreign: Acapulco Gold, Acapulco Red, Angola Black, Bhang, Black Gold, Black Gungeon, Black Gunion, Blue Sky Blond, Cam Red, Cambodian Trip Weed, Canadian Black, Colombian, Conga, Conga Brown, Congo Mataby, Ganja, Gold Leaf, Jamaican, Kona Gold, Leper Grass, Machu Picchu, Maui, Mexican Brown, Mexican Green, Mexican Red, Oaxacan, P.R., Panama Gold, Panama Red, Park Land Number Twos, Punta Roja, Santa Maria Gold, Santa Maria Red, Thai Stick, Thai Weed, Wacky Weed, Wahegan, Zacatecas Purple
Marihuana, high potency: Black Mo, Black Moat, Black Mold, Black Mole, Black Monte, Black Mota, Chiba Chiba, Dynamite, Gold, Gold Leaf, Ice Bag, Ice Pack, One-toke Weed, Pato de gayina, Sess, Sinsemilla, Supremo, Wacky Weed, Whacky Weed
Marihuana, liquid: Oil, One, Son of One. *See also* Hashish Oil
Marihuana, low potency: Bam, Bammies, Bammy, Blank, Bull Jive, Bunk, Dirt Grass, Garbage, Lipton's, Punk, Salt and Pepper
Marihuana, quantities for sale: Bag, Bar, Brick, Box, Can, Deck, Deuce Bag, Dime Bag, Dirty Short, Eighth, Elbow, Fifty Cent Bag, Kee, Key, Ki, Matchbox, Moon, Nickle Bag, Ounce, Piece. *See also* Quantity, drug

Marihuana, To smoke: Bang, Be in Weeds, Beat the Weeds, Bending the Head, Bite One's Lip, Blast, Blow, Blow a Stick, Blow One's Top, Bounce the Goof Balls, Break a Stick, Burn an Indian, Burn the Hay, Bust, Do, Do a Joint, Do Up, Doing your Business, Drag, Drink Texas Tea, Drop a Joint, Fire Up, Get Down, Get it On, Get Off, Get On, Go Loco, Goofing, Hit, Hit the Hay, Hoka Toka, Humping the Sage, In Tweeds, Kiss Mary Jane, Knock Yourself Crazy, Lie in State with the Girls, Light Up, Pick Up, Poke, Poking, Pot Out, Power Hit, Pull, Send, Send Up, Sipping, Smoke Rings, Straighten Out, Taste, Tighten Your Wig, Toak, Toat, Toke, Toke Up, Torch Up, Tote, Trigger, Turkey, Turn On, Twist a Giraffe's Tail, Vipe, Waste

Marihuana cigarette: Ace, Bammies, Bams, Bammy, Bomb, Bomber, Boo Reefer, Booster Stick, Burnies, Butt, Cancelled Stick, Cartucho, Cat Tail, Ceck, Cigar, Cocktail, Dinky Dow, Doped Cigarette, Double Header, Dream Stick, Dynamiters, Fat Jay, Fatty, Fraho, Frajo, Funny Cigarettes, Gage Butt, Gasper, Gauge Butt, Gold Leaf Special, Gonga Smudge, Goober, Goof Butt, Gow, Guage Butt, Gyves, Happy Cigarette, Hay Butt, Hot Stick, Kick Stick, Killer, Killer Stick, Leno, Log, Meserole, Mezz, Mezz Roll, Miggles, Mighty Mezz, Ming, Muggles, Nail, Nose Burner, Nose Warmer, Number, Pack, Panatella, Pin, Pinner, Reefer, Roach, Root, Sass-fras, Seed, Single, Skoofus, Skrufer, Skrufus, Solid, Special, Spliff, Splim, Splint, Stack, Stencil, Stick, Tea Bag, Thing, Thirteen, Thriller, Thumb, Torch, Torpedo, Tube, Twist, Vonce, Zol

Marihuana cigarette papers: Bambu, Banana, Blanco y Negro, Blanket, EZ Wider

Marihuana user: Bambalacha Rambler, Blow Top, Blower, Bo Bo Jockey, Boreroom Beater, Bushwacker, Butt, Dope Head, Doper, Dopester, Fay Hound, Freak, Fu Manchu, Goof, Gouger, Gowster, Grass Eater, Grasshopper, Green, Griefer, Hay Burner, Hay Head, Head, Hop Head, Jane's Better Half, Junkerman, Lover, Lusher, Mugglehead, Oiler, Pot Head, Pot Lush, Reefer Hound, Reefing Man, Roach Bender, Sagebrush Whacker, Tea Blower, Tea Head, Tea Hound, Teo, Texas Leaguer, T-man, Toker, Twister, User, Viper, Weed Eater, Weed Head, Weed Hound, Weed Twister, Weedly, Weekend Doper, Weekend Tripper, Weekend User, Youngblood

Mescaline: Bad Seed, Big Chief, Cactus Button, Football, Mesc, Mescal, Outer, Plants, Pumpkin Seeds, Wakowi, Yellow Footballs, Yellow Submarines. *See also* Peyote

Methadone: Biscuits, Chalk, Collies, Dollies, Dolly, Dolophine, Wafers

Methaqualone: Canadian Quail, Lemmon 714, Lemmons, Lude, Mandrax, Medicine, Optimil, Parest, Quaalude, Quacks, Quad, Quas, Seven-one-fours, Soapers, Soaps, Super Quaaludes, Super Soper, Wallbangers

Money: Abe, Bread, Folding Stuff, Geetis, Lettuce, Lincoln, Long Green, Powdered Bread, Scratch

Morning-glory seeds: Blue Morning, Flying Saucers, Heavenly Blue, Pearly Gates, Pearly Whites, Seeds, Summer Skies, Tlitiltzen, Wedding Bells

Morphine: Acetomorphine, Amilerdine, Bang, Barmecide, Big M, Birdie Powder, Birdie Stuff, Cobies, Coby, Cube, Cube Juice, Em, Emm, Emsel,

Glad Stuff, Goma, Gonga Dust, Happy Medicine, Hard Stuff, Hell Dust, Hocus, Joy Dust, Joy Flakes, M, Marmon, Miss Emma, Miss Emma Jones, Miss Morph, Monkey Morphine, Moocah, Morph, Morphie, Morphina, Morpho, Morphy, Morshtop, Mr. Morpheus, Number Thirteen, Piece, Red Cross, Sister, Sugar, Sweet Jesus, Sweet Morpheus, Tab, Uncle, Unkie, Unkle, White Cross, White Death, White Goddess, White Linen, White Merchandise, White Nurse, White Powder, White Silk, White Stuff, White Tape, Wings, Witch

Narcotics: Acetylmethadol, Alpha Powder, Alphrodine, Arsenal, Bang, Bingle, Birdie Stuff, Bug Juice, Caronotics, Cotics, Demerol, Demis, Dihydrocodeine, Dilaudid, Dillies, Dilocol, Dope, Dreams, Dry Booze, Dry Grog, Easing Powder, Fairy Powder, Feed, Fun Medicine, Ganger, Garbage, Geeser, Geez, Geezer, Goods, Gosneaks, Grog, Happy Dust, Happy Flakes, Happy Powder, Happy Stuff, Hop in Paper, Hot Stuff, Isonipecaine, LAAM, Lady White, Locus, Mahoska, Maude C., Merchandise, Mojo, Mooch, Nocks, Pentazocine, Powdered Joy, Sugar and Salt, Water of Life. *See also* Heroin; Morphine; Narcotics, low potency

Narcotics, low potency: Blanks, Dummy, Flea Powder, Ganger, Garbage, Hot Stuff, Leather Dew, Lemon, Lemonade, Lipton Tea, Nixon, Turkey

Narcotics use, beginning: Breaking In, Cadet, Convert, Fledgling, Freshen, Freshman, Get in the Groove, Get Narkied, Give Him His Wings, Green Hype, Honeymoon, Hoosier, Hoosier Fiend, Laodicean, Needled, Student, Taste Blood

Narcotics user: Ad, Artic Explorer, Bangster, Bindle Kate, Bindle Stiff, Birdcage Hype, Birdhouse Hype, Cotton Head, Cotton Picker, Cotton Shooter, Cotton Top, Creep, Crowd, Dope Fiend, Dope Fighter, Dope Hop, Drug Partisan, Eater, Feeblo, Fledgling, Flier, Gal Head, Gowhead, Gowster, Hop Head, Hopper, Hoppie, Hops Stiff, Hopster, Hype, Junker, Junkie, Pasty Face, Prodder, Racehorse Charlie, R.F.D. Junker, Safety Pin Mechanic, Saturday Nighter, Sleepwalker, Smack Head, Smokey, Stoner, Sun in the Moons, Tecato. *See also* Addict

Nembutal: Abbotts, Canary, Nembees, Nemish, Nemmy, Nimby, Yellow Angels, Yellow Birds, Yellow Bullets, Yellow Jackets, Yellows. *See also* Barbiturates

Nitrous oxide: Laughing Gas, Whippets

Non–drug-user: Apple, Brown Shoes, Do-Righter, John, Lame Duck, Square, Square Apple, Straight

Opium: Auntie, Big O, Black Pill, Black Shit, Black Snake, Black Stuff, Brew Units, Brick Gum, Brown Hash, Brown Stuff, Bunk, Button, Chicory, Chinese Molasses, Chocolate, Cookie Mud, Cutered Pill, Dopium, Dream, Dream Beads, Dream Wax, Elevation, Fire-Plug, Foon, Fun, Ghow, Glad Stuff, Goma, Gow, Gow Crust, Goynk, Grease, Green Ashes, Green Mud, Green Powder, Gum, Ice Cream, K.O.'s, Laudanum, Leaf Gum, Lemkee, Li Un, Li Yuen, Lightning Smoke, Mahogany Juice, Midnight Oil, Molasses, Munsh, O, Op, Pan Juice, Pan Yen, Pekoe, Pellicle, Pen Yen,

Piki, Pill, Pillow, Poppy, Poppy Rain, Poppy Train, Pox, P.S., Puff, Rooster Brand, Root Tonic, Sam How, San Lo, Scours, Sealing Wax, Son Lo, Tar, Yen Chee, Yen Chiang, Yen Pock, Yen Shee, Yen Shee Suey. *See also* Narcotics

Opium use: Beat the Gong, Burn the Midnight Oil, Chef, Cook, Cook a Pill, Cooker, Deep Breath Spasms, Flop, Get Yen, Going to the Laundry, Hit the Gong, Hit the Pipe, Hit the Stem, In Dreams, Kick the Gong, Kick the Pipe Around, Kick the Rag, Kick the Toy, Lay against the Engine, Lay Down, Lay the Stem, Lie on Your Hip, Melt Wax, Puff on the Side, Puffing, Riding the Pipe, Roll in Black Stuff, Roll the Boy, Roll the Log, Slapping the Bamboo, Smoking the Pipe, Suck Bamboo

Paraldehyde: Parackie, Paral, Paraldy

Paraphernalia, amphetamine: B bomb, Crystal ship

Paraphernalia, cocaine: Cocaine Kit, Dessicator, Ether Base, Freebase Conversion Kit, Nasal Irrigator, Shaker Jar, Winky

Paraphernalia, marihuana: Acapulco Gold Papers, Airplane, Bambu, Bambu Case, Blanco y Negro, Blanket, Bong, Bridge, Carburetor, Chillum, Clip, Cock Pipe, Crutch, CWP, Dope Pipe, E-Z Wider, Grass Pipe, Hash Cannon, Head Gear, Head Shop, Hookah, Hubble Bubble, Jay Pipe, Jefferson Airplane, Marfil, Papers, Rizla, Roach Clip, Rolling Machine, Rolling Paper, Shotgun, Sifter, Slave Master, Stash Container, Steam Roller, Steamboat, Stella, Toke Pipe, Top, Water Pipe, Wheaties, Zig Zag, Zig Zag Man, Zooie, Z-kit

Paraphernalia, narcotics: Artillery, Bay State, Bayonet, Biz, Boo-gee, Cannon, Collar, Cook, Cooker, Cooking Spoon, Cotton, Dinghiyen, Dingus, Dope Gun, Dripper, Dropper, Energy Gun, Engine, Factory, Fake, Fake Aloo, Fit, G, Gasket, Gimmicks, Glass, Glass Gun, Gun, Hard Nail, Harpoon, Hit Spike, Hop Gun, Horse and Wagon, Hype Stick, Ickey, Job's Antidote, Johnson and Johnson, Joint, Kit, Layout, Light Artillery, Luer, Machine, Machinery, Monkey Drill, Monkey Pump, Mr. Twenty-Six, Nail, Needle, Outfit, Pin Gun, Point, Prick, Quill, Rig, Safety, Satch Cotton, Set, Sharps, Spike, Spike and Dripper, Spike and Jolt, Spoon, Stabber, Tie, Tools, Works, Yale

Paraphernalia, opium: Altar, Chinese Saxophone, Death Needle, Dream Pipe, Dream Stick, Gee Bag, Gee Gee, Gee Rag, Gee Stick, Gee Yen, Geep, Gong, Gonger, Gongkicker, Gongola, Hop Stick, Hop Toy, Humming Bowl, Humming Gee Bowl, Joy Stick, Layette, Layout, Lemmon Bowl, Log, Log Stick, Pig, Pop Stick, Saddle and Bridle, Saxophone, Stein, Stem, Suey Pow, Toy, Yen Gow, Yen Hock, Yen Hoke

Paregoric: Blue Velvet, Goric, P.G., P.O., Proctor and Gamble

PCP: Ace, Ad, Amoeba, Angel Dust, Angel Hair, Angel Mist, Angel Puke, Animal, Animal Tranquilizer, Aurora Borealis, Black Whack, Busy Bee, Cadillac, Cigarrode Cristal, CJ, Columbo, Cozmos, Cristal, Crystal, Crystal Points, Crystal T, Cyclones, Detroit Pink, Devil Dust, Dime of Buzz, Dipper, DOA, Dummy Dust, Dust, Dust of Angels, Earth, Elephant, Elephant Tranquilizer, Embalming Fluid, Energizer, Fake STP, Flake, Fuel, Goon, Goon Dust, Gorilla Tab, Green, Green Tea, Heaven and Hell, Herms, Heroin Buzz, Hog, Horse Tranquilizer, Jet Fuel, Juice, K, K-blast, Kaps, Ketamine, Killerweed, KJ Crystal, Kools, KW, Live Ones, Lovely Magic, Magic, Magic Dust, Mean Green, Mintweed, Mist, Monkey Dust, More, New Magic, Niebla, Orange Crystal, Ozone, P, Parsley, PAZ, PCPA, Peace, Peace Pill, Peaceweed, Peanut Butter, Peter Pan, Pig Killer, Polvo, Polvo de Angel, Product IV, Puffy, Rocket Fuel, Scaffle, Sernyl, Sheets, Shermans, Sherms, Smoking Snorts, Soma, Spores, Star Dust, Stick, Super, Super Joint, Super Kools, Super Rass, Super Weed, Surfer, Synthetic Cocaine, Synthetic Marihuana, Synthetic THC, T, Tac, T-buzz, Tea, THC, TIC, Tic-Tac, Trank, TT-1, TT-2, TT-3, Water, Weed, Whack Wack, White Powder, Wobble Weed, Wolf, Worm, Yellow Fever, Zombie Buzz, Zoom

Pentobarbital sodium: *See* Nembutal

Percodan: Percobarb, Percs, Perks

Peyote: Button, Cactus, Full Moon, Hikori, Mescal Beans, Mescal Buttons, P, Semi, Top, Topi, Tops. *See also* Mescaline

Phenobarbital: Luminal, Phenies, Pheno, Purple Hearts, Whites

Physician: Croaker, Dr. Feelgood, Ice Tong Doctor, Ice Water John, Right Croaker

Police: Big John, Bim, Black and White, Blue Fascist, Bull, Buster, Cop, Crusher, Deadwood, Dope Cop, Fed, Fuzz, Gazer, G-man, Heat, Lard, Nabs, Nailers, Narc, Narcotic Bulls, Pig, Sam, Snoops, The Man, T-man, Uncle, Whiskers

Possession, drug: Anywhere, Carrying, Dirty, Fat, Holding, Squirrel

Preparation, marihuana: Clean, Cure, Cut, Gage in the Rough, Lumber, Manicure, Mud, Roll, Shake, Stretch, Tuck and Roll, Twist a Dream

Prescription: Monkey with a Long Tail, Monkey with a Short Tail, Paper, Per, Reader, Reader with a Long Tail, Reader with a Short Tail, Script, Script with a Tail

Psilocybin: Noble Princess of the Waters, Shrooms, Silly Putty

Quantity, drug: Bag, Bale of Hay, Balloon, Bar, Big Hog, Bird's Eye, Bindle, Biz, Block Box, Bottle, Brick, Can, Cap, Card, Cargo, Cube, Deck, Deuce, Deuce Bag, Dime Bag, Elbow, Feed Bag, Finger, Foil, Full Moon, Gang, Gram, Half, Half Bundle, Half Load, Half Piece, Hunk, Jug, Kee, Keg, Key, Ki, Kite, Ky, Lid, Load, Long, Match, Matchbox, Matchhead, Microgram, Milligram, Moon, Nickel, Nickel Bag, O, Ohio Bag, O.Z., Paper, Piece, Pillow, Quarter Bag, Quarter Ounce, Sack, Short, Short Piece, Sixteenth, Spoon, Tens, Tin, Z. *See also:* Marihuana, quantities for sale

Religious use, of marihuana: Boo Hoo, Nepalese Temple Balls, Nepalese Temple Hash, Rastafarianas, Soma

Residual effects: Ear Rings, Echoes, Flashback

Seconal: Apple, Bala, Blunt, Canadian Bouncer, F-Forties, F-Sixty-sixes, Gum Drop, Mand M's, Marshmallow Reds, Mexican Reds, Pink Ladies, Pinks,

Pula, R.D.'s, Red Birds, Red Bullets, Red Devils, Red Dolls, Red Jack-
    ets, Red Lillies, Reds, Sec, Seccies, Secy, Seggies, Seggy. *See also* Bar-
    biturates
Smuggling: Body Packing, Dope Ring, Jail Plant, Keester Plant, Mule, Pack
    One's Keyster, Put it in Writing, Rubber Pill, Wire

Tranquilizers: Backwards, Chlordiazepoxide, Chlorpromazine, Diazepam,
    Downers, Downs, Equanil, Miltown, Muscle Relaxer, Neuroleptic, Ox-
    azepam, Tranks, Tranqs, Valium. *See also* Barbiturates
Tuinal: Double Trouble, F-sixty-sixes, Rainbow, Reds and Blues, Tooies, Toot-
    sie, Trees, Tuies

Under the influence, of a drug: A Boot, All Lit Up, Amok, Amuck, Backed
    Up, Basted, Be Sent, Beaming, Bean Trip, Belted, Bent, Bent Out of
    Shape, Blasted, Blind, Blitzed, Blocked, Bombed, Boxed, Buzz, Buzzed,
    Call, Cap Out, Charge, Climes on you, Cloud Nine, Coasting, Coked Up,
    Contact High, Cooked Up, Crazy, Delirium, Dope Jag, Dragged, Drunk,
    Feathered, Fired, Flattened, Flip, Floating, Flying, Flying in the Clouds,
    Foxy, Fractured, Frazzled, Fried to the Gills, Frosted, Frosty Frozen,
    Frozen, Full Blast, Full of Junk, Fuzzy, Goofed, Gowed, Gowed Up,
    Grifado, Halvahed, Heaped, High, Hit the Moon, Horsed, In, In a Nod,
    In Flight, In Orbit, In the Air, In Transit, Jacked Up, Jag, Jailhouse
    High, Jolt, Joy Ride, Keyed Up, Kick, Laughing Jag, Leaping and
    Stinking, Leaps, Lit Up, Loaded, Muggled Up, Nodding, Numbered Out,
    On, On the Nod, Ossified, Overamped, Overcharged, Overdosed, Packed
    Up, Passed Out, Polluted, Poppied, Pottledripped, Purring Like a Kit-
    ten, Ripped, Rolling Buzz, Running Amok, Rush, Set on His Ass, Seven-
    foot Step, Shot Up, Sleigh Riding, Spaced Out, Stoned, Straight, Tall,
    Tead Up, There, Torn Up, Trip, Turned On, Up, Wiped Out, Wired,
    Zipped, Zonked. *See also* Exhaustion, due to drug use; High
Units, drug: *See* Quantity, drug

Withdrawal, narcotic: Abstinence, Abstinence Syndrome, Agonies, Cat Nap,
    Catch Up, Clear Up, Feel the Thing Coming On, Fold Up, Got it Beat,
    Hang Up, Kick, Kipping, Make the Turn, Take the Boil Out, Take the
    Cure, Three-Day Habit, Whips and Jingles, Wormy, Yenning. *See also*
    Abstinence, drug
Withdrawal, narcotic, abrupt: Boil Out Cure, Cold Turkey, Hang Tough, Ice
    Water Cure, Iron Cure, Kick Cold, Make it Steel and Concrete, On the
    Natch, Quarry Cure, Rock Pile Cure, Sneeze it Out, Steel and Concrete
    Cure, Steel Cure, Sweat Cure
Withdrawal, narcotic, feigned: Brody, Bug, Cartwheel, Chuck a Wingding,
    Circus, Clown, Do a Figure Eight, Do an Inger, Make a Croaker for a
    Reader, Meter, Play the Clown, Put on a Circus, Put the Croaker On,
    Put the Croaker to Work, Throw a Brody, Throw a Meter, Throw a
    Wingding, Turn a Cartwheel, Turn on the Wobbler, Wing Ding, Wob-
    bler.

Withdrawal, narcotic, gradual: Bend the Needle, Rat-tail Cure, Sissy Cure, Slack-off Cure, Taper-off Cure

Withdrawal sickness: Abstinence Syndrome, Agonies, Around the Bend, Be Sick, Be Washed Up, Chinaman's Dance, Fourth Degree, Frontier, Going Downhill, Chinaman on (one's) Back, Monkey on (one's) Back, Himmelsbach Test, Hurting, In Trouble, Junk Stage, Monkey Scratch, Over the Hump, Reach the Pitch, Scratching, Sickness, Sweat it Out, Twisted

Bibliography

Abel, E. L. *A Marihuana Dictionary*. Westport, Conn.: Greenwood Press, 1982.

Algren, N. *The Man with the Golden Arm*. New York: Doubleday and Co., 1949.

Anonymous. "A hashish house in New York." *Harper's New Monthly Magazine* 67 (1883): 944–49.

Anslinger, H. J. "Marihuana: Assassin of Youth." *American Magazine* 124 (1937): 18–19, 150–53.

Anslinger, H. J., and Tompkins, W. F. *The Traffic in Narcotics*. New York: Funk and Wagnalls Co., 1953.

Berrey, L. V., and Van den Bark, M. *The American Thesaurus of Slang: A Complete Reference Book of Colloquial Speech*. New York: Thomas Y. Crowell, 1942.

Black, W. *Dope: The Story of the Living Dead*. New York: Star Co., 1928.

Bloomquist, E. R. *Marihuana* Beverly Hills, Calif.: Glencoe Press, 1968.

Braddy, H. "Narcotic Argot along the Mexican Border." *American Speech* 30 (1955): 84–90.

———. "The Anonymous Verses of a Narcotic Addict." *Southern Folklore Quarterly*, September 1958, pp. 130–38.

Brennan, M. *Drugs*. San Antonio: Naylor Co., 1970.

Brown, C. *Manchild in the Promised Land*. New York: Macmillan Co., 1965.

Burroughs, W. S. *Junkie*. New York: Ace Books, 1953.

———. *Naked Lunch*. New York: Grove Press, 1959.

Claerbaut, D. *Black Jargon in White America*. New York: Wm. B. Erdman, 1972.

Cooper, C. R. *Here's to Crime*. Boston: Little, Brown, and Co., 1937.

Coyote Man. *Get the Buzz On*. Berkeley: Brother William Press, 1972.

Cromwell, P. F. "Slang Usage in the Addict Subculture." *Journal of Drug Issues* 1 (1970): 75–78.

Danforth, H. R., and Horan, J. D. *Big City Crimes*. New York: Permabooks, 1957.

De Lannoy, W. C., and Masterson, E. "Teen-age Hophead Jargon." *American Speech* 27 (1952): 23–31.

DeLeeuw, H. *Flower of Joy*. New York: Lee Furman, 1939.

De Lenoir, C. *The Hundredth Man*. New York: Clauden Kendall, 1934.

Donovan, J. A. "Jargon of Marihuana Addicts." *American Speech* 15 (1940): 336–37.

Folb, E. A. "A Comparative Study of Urban Black Argot." Ph.D. diss., University of California, Los Angeles, 1972.

Geller, A., and Boas, M. *The Drug Beat*. New York: Cowles Book Co., 1969.

Goldin, H. E.; O'Leary, F.; and Lipsius, M. *Dictionary of American Underworld Lingo*. New York: Twayne Publishing Co., 1950.

Goldman, A. *Grass Roots*. New York: Warner Books, 1980.

Gomerly, S. *Drugs and the Canadian Scene*. Toronto: Burns and Macechern, 1970.

Gottschalk, L. A., and Cowdry, F. W. "The Language of the Narcotic Addict." Paper presented at the United States Public Health Service Hospital, Fort Worth, 1948.

Hardy, R., and Cull, J. G. *Drug Language and Lore*. Springfield, Ill.: C. C. Thomas, 1975.

Harney, M. L., and Cross, J. C. *The Narcotic Officer's Notebook*. Springfield, Ill.: C. C. Thomas, 1973.

Harris, J. D. *The Junkie Priest*. New York: Pocket Books, 1965.

Heard, N. C. *Howard Street*. New York: Dial Press, 1968.

Herron, D. M., and Anderson, L. F. *Can We Survive Drugs?*. Philadelphia: Chilton Book Co., 1970.

Himes, C. *For Love of Imabelle*. New York: Signet Books, 1965.

Holiday, B. *Lady Sings the Blues*. New York: Lancer Books, 1959.

Howsley, L. B. *Argot: A Dictionary of Underworld Slang*. Seattle: Columbia Publishing Co., 1935.

Hughes, H. M. *The Fantastic Lodge*. Boston: Houghton Mifflin Co., 1961.

Iceberg Slim. *Pimp: The Story of My Life*. Los Angeles: Holloway House Publishing Co., 1969.

La Guardia Committee on Marihuana. *The Marihuana Problem in the City of New York*. Metuchen, N. J.: Scarecrow Reprint Corp., 1973.

Lait, J., and Mortimer, L. *Washington Confidential*. New York: Dell Publishing Co., 1951.

Lentini, J. R. *Vice and Narcotics Control*. Beverly Hills, Calif.: Glencoe Press, 1977.

Lindesmith, A. "The Argot of the Underworld Drug Addict." *Journal of Criminal Law and Criminology* 29 (1938): 261–78.

———. *Addiction and Opiates*. Chicago: Aldine Publishing Co., 1968.

Lipton, L. *The Holy Barbarians*. New York: Grove Press, 1959.

Mandell, G. *Flee the Angry Strangers*. New York: Bobbs-Merrill Co., 1952.

Maurer, D. W. "The Argot of the Underworld Narcotic Addict." *American Speech* 11 (1936): 116–27.

———. "The Argot of the Underworld Narcotic Addict: Part II." *American Speech* 11 (1936): 179–92.

———. "Speech of the Narcotic Underworld." *American Mercury* 62 (1946): 225–30.

———. "Marijuana Addicts and Their Lingo." *American Mercury* 63 (1946): 571–76.

Maurer, D. W., and Vogel, V. H. *Narcotics and Narcotic Addiction*. Springfield, Ill.: C. C. Thomas, 1973.

Mencken, H. L. *The American Language*. Supplement 2. New York: Alfred A. Knopf, 1962.

Mezzrow, M., and Wolfe, B. *Really the Blues*. New York: Dell Publishing Co., 1946.

Novak, W. *High Culture*. New York: Alfred A. Knopf, 1980.

Partridge, E. A. *A Dictionary of the Underworld*. New York: Bonanza Books, 1961.

PharmChem Newsletter. 1980–1981. Menlo Park, Calif.

Pollock, A. *The Underworld Speaks*. San Francisco: Prevent Crime Bureau, 1935.

Preble, E., and Casey, J.J. "Taking Care of Business—The Heroin User's Life on the Street." *International Journal of the Addictions* 4 (1969): 1–24.

Pritchie, N. *The Savage Kick*. New York: Fawcett Books, 1962.

Schmidt, J. E. *Narcotics, Lingo and Lore*. Springfield, Ill.: C. C. Thomas, 1959.

Selby, H. *Last Exit to Brooklyn*. New York: Grove Press, 1957.

Siegel, R. K. "Cocaine Smoking." *Journal of Psychoactive Drugs* 14 (1982): 271–359.

Siragusa, C. *The Trail of the Poppy*. Englewood Cliffs, N. J.: Prentice-Hall, 1966.

Smith, D. E., and Gray, G. R. *It's So Good, Don't Even Try It Once*. Englewood Cliffs, N. J.: Prentice-Hall, 1972.

Sullivan, J. M. *Criminal Slang*. Boston: Underworld Publishing Co., 1908.

Thomas, P. *Down These Mean Streets*. New York: Signet Books, 1967.

Trocchi, A. *Cain's Book*. New York: Grove Press, 1961.

Wells, W. H. "Words Used in Drug Traffic." *Dialect Notes* 1 (1922): 181–82.

Wentworth, H., and Fexner, S. B. *Dictionary of American Slang*. New York: Thomas Y. Crowell, 1975.

Westin, A., and Shaffer, S. *Heroes and Heroin*. New York: Pocket Books, 1972.

Woodley, R. *Dealer*. New York: Holt, Rinehart, and Winston, 1971.

Young, L. A.; Young, L. G.; Klein, M. M.; Klein, D. M.; and Beyer, D. *Recreational Drugs*. New York: Collier Books, 1977.

About the Author

ERNEST L. ABEL is a Research Scientist at the Research Institute on Alcoholism in Buffalo, New York. His other works include *Narcotics and Reproduction* (1983), *Drugs and Sex* (1983), *Alcohol and Reproduction* (1982), and *Smoking and Reproduction* (1982), all published by Greenwood Press.